"This is one family's story about the unbearable tragedy of AIDS. One of the early victims in this epidemic, Ralph Newman, acquired HIV from a blood transfusion, before blood could be screened as it now is. It is a heart-breaking story, but one that reflects the courage of a family that was not resigned, but which sought all avenues of care, all possibilities for palliation or cure. The Newman family should take great pride in the their efforts to ease Ralph's suffering and to ensure that society take the necessary steps to minimize other families being in similar circumstances."

Martin J. Blaser, M.D.
President-elect, Infectious Diseases Society of America
May 15, 2005
New York University School of Medicine

It has been over 20 years since Mr. Ralph Newman and family walked through my office door. That day was like any other, but the Newman family was not. What I remember most about this remarkable family was the determination of Mr. Newman to get to the bottom line diagnosis to solve this medical mystery. The logic and inquisitive nature of his engineering mind drove him to seek answers and solutions that were often beyond our capabilities at that time. His determination inspired me to do all that was humanly possible. I was equally awestruck by the love and support of his family. Like Mr. Newman, they were equally curious and more often than not, we did not have the answers to their questions. My experience with Mr. Newman and family has left me with some lifelong lessons. Foremost of these, are the importance of family love and support, and the indomitable influence of spirit in carrying on in face of a terminal diagnosis.

Mr. Newman's Physician
Mayo Clinic
Rochester, MN

TOMORROW WE'LL KNOW

A True Story

by

Beverly M. Newman

authorHOUSE™

1663 LIBERTY DRIVE, SUITE 200
BLOOMINGTON, INDIANA 47403
(800) 839-8640
WWW.AUTHORHOUSE.COM

First published by AuthorHouse 10/26/05

ISBN: 1-4208-6354-1 (sc)

Library of Congress Control Number: 2005905703

Printed in the United States of America
Bloomington, Indiana

This book is printed on acid-free paper.

****

Although the names of Dr. Morrow and Dr. Fraser are fictitious, their roles as compassionate, understanding individuals are real. They trudged the lonely path with us sharing our hopes and fears. We shall always be grateful to them.

****

Cover Design by Patrick Mallek
Mallek Creative
Boulder, Colorado

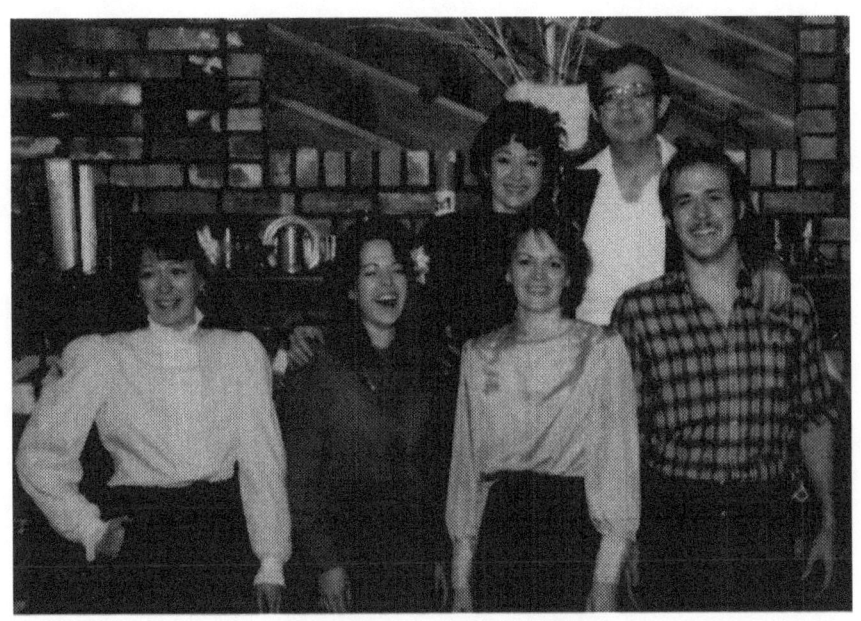

New Year's Eve 1983-1984
Rachelle, Kathy, Laurie, R.P.
Beverly and Ralph

To my children –
For the love they shared.

For their children –
So they will always know.

Today's almost over –
No answers in sight.
There's always tomorrow –
Don't give up the fight!

Tomorrow's the answer!
That's what we say.
It's the hope and the promise
Of one brand new day.

So chase all those rainbows,
Search, work and grow.
Thank God for the promise,
Tomorrow We'll Know!

Rachelle Newman Mollohan

Prologue

Ralph never saw his enemy. For more than two years, he wrestled and struggled with his insidious foe, until the embattled warrior lay weak and wasted, his cunning enemy entrenched and indestructible. The evil, haughty laughter of the victor may have been discernible in the room were it not for the rhythmic gurgling of the aspirator tube in Ralph's rib cage.

Bev hit the window with her fist. "Damn you! You ugly monster! You're going to win!" she cried, tears of hurt fear and anger streaming down her face. The vastness of the city with its millions of tiny flickering lights failed to spark the excitement as it had five years before. Ralph's battle and the taunting of his clever enemy had dulled her senses and corroded her spirit.

She looked back across the dimly lit room. The "troops" were huddled around the bed planning another maneuver. Ralph had fought the front line, but his tiny platoon had been behind him supporting him with every weapon at their disposal. Now they were bruised and bloodied from the battle. The fear of impending defeat reflected in their eyes but not one was willing to surrender. They refused to speak of defeat. Their leader had taught them well.

R.P. moved around the end of the bed, snapped up the clipboard to record Ralph's temperature and stood waiting for Laurie to provide him with the pulse rate. The piece of paper towel on the clipboard was a crude substitute for a patient's chart.

"It's the only way we'll know what's happening," Laurie said as she held her fingers to Ralph's wrist to check his pulse rate.

Rachelle knelt down at the side of the bed to determine the flow rate of the lung aspirator as Kathy prepared to open another lemon swab to moisten Ralph's parched lips and tongue.

"We're going to watch Star Trek with you tonight, Dad," Kathy said, hoping for a response. He had been in a coma before and rallied, "It could happen again," she thought.

Ralph's enemy had led them through some rough terrain. They had been conditioned to the peaks and valleys of the path they had trod. Kathy was convinced there would be another peak.

"Can you squeeze my hand, Dad?" she asked, as she held his hand in hers. She looked up at Bev and felt the need to explain his lack of response, "He just needs to sleep now," she said, trying to sooth Bev's hurt as much as her own.

"Mom, why don't you go home and rest tonight, we'll be here to take care of Dad," Rachelle said.

"Yes, I'll go home, but not right now. I'll just go up to the waiting room for a little while," Bev said, not wanting to go home. She had shared home with Ralph for 33 years. He had been her protection from the cold chill of the northwest wind and she shivered at the thought of being alone without that barrier, without his love.

"Please, God, don't let Ralph have any more seizures," she prayed, "He has suffered enough. Just let the medication work now. I'm not going to ask you to make him well. That can't be part of your plan for him. I know I have to accept his dying, but please, just don't let him have any more seizures."

Bev felt relieved. "I'm not asking for a miracle," she thought, "just a little mercy. Ralph is a good person. God is surely aware of his faith.

God may view mine as a little sketchy at times, but not Ralph's. If God won't do this for me, He will for Ralph."

She was relaxed when Kathy entered the waiting room. "Dad's doing okay, Mom," she said, "I just came to tell you so you wouldn't be worrying."

"Thanks, Kath," Bev said, with a smile. She felt stable and calm. "No one has been able to tell us why Daddy is in a coma, have they?"

"Not yet, but Laurie has her medical book here and she's coming in to read whatever she can find."

Laurie walked into the room, the thick book tucked under her arm. She flipped it open to a marked page, sat down between Bev and Kathy and the three proceeded to read.

"This is all the information I can find that fits Dad's case. We know that the white patches in his digestive tract have inhibited absorption of nutrients. A deficiency in vitamin B2 can cause some of Dad's central nervous system symptoms. Let's ask the doctor to give him 200mg of Thiamine daily," Laurie said.

Bev nodded, "Okay. We have nothing to lose."

The three of them exchanged glances and began to laugh. "The doctor will probably call down to the pharmacy and say, 'Hey Charlie, you know what those Newman kooks want now?' but it could work and we have to try," Kathy said.

"I am so glad you kids are here," Bev said, "because we all have to get some rest, but we can't leave Daddy here alone after what happed the last time...."

"You better come right away," Rachelle said as she ran into the waiting room. "Dad's having another seizure!"

"What?!!" I don't believe this!" Bev cried as they ran toward Ralph's room.

Bev rushed to Ralph's bedside. She couldn't look at his face. She stared momentarily at his legs jerking under the bedclothes, and reacted. The object nearest to her, a metal hospital chair, went flying against the wall.

"I asked Him for just one thing!" she cried, "Just one thing, and He couldn't even grant me that!" Shaking from head to foot with pure anger, she felt betrayed by Ralph's God.

Kathy stepped forth to hug and calm her. Bev was not ready to be calmed. She pushed Kathy away and stood alone angrily protesting the seizures.

The nurse put her arm around Bev, "Now, honey, you know there is only so much medical science can do."

"To hell with medical science! I know they can't do anything; I'm talking about Him! She cried, gesturing upward. "He could do something! What does He want? Another pound of flesh? There's nothing left."

They were caught up in a war of global proportions. A war in which only the enemy survives. The deadly invader selects his victims at random and multiplies in the face of their defenses. Unlike the wars man has known throughout history, women and children are not excluded from the battlefront and international law does not apply. The realization that the enemy has touched their shoulder comes slowly and painfully to the victims. Ralph was no exception.

Chapter One

A Sparkling Arch, the colors glow
Above the land and far below,
We stand in wonder,
Stand in awe.
Behold!
The Grandeur
The Mystery
The Law.

Rachelle Newman Mollohan

It was March 1983. Bev and Ralph sat at the coffee table in the corner of their bedroom, a place reserved for sharing peaceful moments while they enjoyed the view of the Rocky Mountain foothills. Now they were bewildered. Ralph's healthy, tan skin had taken on a grayish look with deep lines. The result of a 40 pound weight loss and two months of unexplained fever often accompanied by chills. The doctors they had consulted included a specialist in every field where they felt a problem might exist; none had been successful in defining his illness.

Each morning during those months they awakened with the hope that the tests to be performed would provide an answer and there would be a course of action. However, they had no answers, test

1

results had been essentially negative. They could not give up, but they did not know what to do or where they would go next.

It was unlike Ralph to be so passive. All his life he had been a hard-hitting, straight-down-the-middle, call a spade-a-spade sort of person. If one could karate-chop with words, Ralph could do it. He was the stereotype of an engineer, never without a pocket full of pencils, everything had to compute, be either black or white and he wanted everything around him, including people, to function like well-oiled machines. An aggressive extrovert, he was a natural-born leader. If he was going to participate, he wanted to be the director. Even at 53, he still had an athletic build, altogether a handsome man whose enthusiasm for life had not faded until the past few weeks. Anyone who met Ralph would remember him—not all would like him—but he always made a lasting impression.

Where decisive action came so easily before, now he sat placidly waiting for Bev to make another suggestion. Her shoulders sagged at the thought of the burden. She had no suggestions. "What is happing to us?" she thought. She longed to escape the emotional devastation, to go back to the time when life was simple and good, back to the "crossroads in their life", back to January 1980.....

They had taken their first extended vacation in their 28 years of marriage. They had both worked for the 13 years they had lived in North Dakota. A certain stagnation had set in. They arranged for four weeks of vacation time. The principal purpose of this trip would be assessment of employment opportunities for engineers. Ralph was a registered professional engineer and at the age of 50, with their four children grown, they agreed exploration of the job market was a wise decision.

Their first destination was the Edgar Cayce Foundation in Virginia Beach. This would be a bit of a pilgrimage, primarily Ralph's desire. He felt that somehow he would receive guidance there - spiritual guidance as well as clarification of purpose. It was a rewarding experience. They became absorbed in the writings, dream analysis and parapsychology. Ralph became a staunch believer in reincarnation and the philosophy that one must serve a karma in this life to compensate for erring in the past lives. Through the serving on one's karma, there would be a resulting spiritual development bringing him closer to the Lord.

After three days of relaxation, walking on the beach and enjoying the fresh seafood, they left for Atlanta. Ralph had a special feeling for the Old South having been stationed there during military service. It was fascinating to Bev. They bought notebooks and began recording their dreams, an exercise suggested by Edgar Cayce to promote more open communication between the conscious and the subconscious mind.

These days were so special they often expressed hope that they could visit there again. They were destined to return, but under circumstances even their subconscious minds could not comprehend.

During the course of the vacation, Ralph found the demand for engineers even greater than he had imagined. As a result of an interview with Martin Marietta in Denver, Colorado, he was given an offer of employment in the Aerospace Division.

They discussed the possibility of relocation with their children. Rachelle and Laurie were in favor of the move as was Kathy, though she was devastated at the thought of their leaving North Dakota.

"I don't want you to move, Dad, but you have no choice....I'll miss you so much, but you have no choice," Kathy said.

R.P., (Ralph Paul, Jr.) was the most decisive. "Don't waste any more time, accept the offer and go!"

He accepted the offer and looked forward to the new challenge.

Ralph and Bev were excited about starting life in a new location. Rachelle and Jim lived in Denver and Ralph and Bev were pleased to be near them and for the opportunity to see more of their grandchildren, Brian, 4 and Jill, 1.

Ralph selected a new home while Bev was still in North Dakota. They were happy with the most beautiful house they had ever owned. It was much larger than they needed, but Ralph was determined he would have a home that would accommodate their entire family when they came to visit.

"I will call this Shiloh—a haven for the whole family," he said.

This was the beginning of the "golden days". The companionship they experienced during the five months to follow was like a reward for all the years of struggle. They would go shopping, buy something new for the house, come home and work with youthful enthusiasm. As soon as the days turned cool, they took delight in lighting the fireplace. They had waited 20 years for a fireplace. It all seemed so perfect. It would have been nice to hold each day in the palm of the hand so they could enjoy it again at will.

Chapter Two

Prior to the arrival of their first weekend guests in early November 1980, Ralph had experienced a week of extreme fatigue, but he was determined his stereo would be operational.

"A house is not a home until it has a good sound system," he said.

It was necessary to pull wires through the crawl space to allow the speakers to be properly placed. While he was under the floor making the initial evaluation, the first pain hit. He came upstairs, his face flushed, the pulse throbbing in his throat.

"Leave the speakers where they are. It's not that important," Bev said.

"It is that important! I'm going to do this today!"

He returned to the crawl space, only to have the pain in his chest hit again. Bev did not wish to upset him further by insisting that he abandon his project. She strung the wires through at his direction, finishing one hour before their guests arrived.

The fatigue persisted through the weekend and on Monday morning; Bev made an appointment with an internist, who had him in an ambulance on the way to the hospital within an hour. The cardiogram had been suspicious and the doctor chose not to take any chances.

He was a young doctor who Bev knew at first sight could be easily intimidated by Ralph in his usual form. However, Ralph accepted the doctor's advice with a minimal amount of grumbling.

Ralph was placed in the coronary care unit where there were no windows, no bathroom privileges and constant monitoring. He called it the "penal colony".

He pushed and prodded the doctors to get on with the tests as he knew the problem was his stomach. He wanted to get to a room where he could look out the window and have a cigarette when he wanted one.

All tests for digestive disturbance were negative. The doctors still thought there was a problem with his heart. Ralph badgered the doctors for the necessary tests to rule in or rule out a heart condition, using his best bulldog tactics. The doctors did their best to humor him, be congenial and at the same time provide the proper medical care.

A stress test was done isolating the problem to the heart. An angiogram was recommended.

When Laurie and Kathy heard of the scheduled angiogram, they arranged their trip to Denver. Laurie, with her new husband, Tom, and Kathy arrived a few hours before the scheduled procedure. They were unprepared for the scene they encountered. The angiogram had been cancelled and Ralph was being transferred back to coronary unit.

"What happened?" Laurie asked as they hurriedly gathered Ralph's personal belongings.

"About 30 minutes ago Daddy had what appears to be a heart attack. The doctors will not be sure until tomorrow morning, but they are reasonably certain there has been heart damage," Bev said.

"Oh, no! God, Mom, he is so young, Laurie said.

"I'm going to call Steve," Kathy said, "I know he'll want to be here. He can bring Stephanie. I want Dad to see her. She's grown so much."

"Would you call R.P. too? He could catch a flight after classes today," Bev said.

Ralph was sedated and returned to the "penal colony". The doctor scheduled insertion of a balloon pump to reduce the backpressure on the heart and relieve the pain.

Though R.P. knew this was a critical time to be away from classes, he came in on the late flight that night. His instructors at the University of North Dakota were very understanding, but as a result of time lost, some of the heavy engineering courses had to be dropped and picked up the next semester. R.P. never regretted coming to Denver that night.

When Steve and Stephanie arrived the next day, all of Ralph's family was with him. Steve and Laurie had been in college together and both had degrees in Medical Technology. Their knowledge of test procedures and familiarity with hospital jargon gave everyone a feeling of security. The day before Thanksgiving 1980, triple coronary bypass surgery was performed.

In his drug-induced, half-conscious twilight before surgery, Ralph had a vision of someone looking like his grandmother, gentle and kind, smiling at him. She was dressed in black wearing a witch's hat. An insignificant dream? Or a symbolic paradoxical vision.

"You will be allowed to see him for a few minutes after surgery, but he won't respond until tomorrow," the doctor said.

After seven hours, Ralph was brought from surgery through the corridor lined on both sides by his family. A muffled cheer went up as he passed by opening his eyes and raising his hand in vague acknowledgement of their presence.

"His heart is very strong," the doctor said, smiling. "As a matter of fact, we had a difficult time getting it to stop beating when we put him on the heart and lung machine."

"That's Dad," R.P. said, "It takes more than heart surgery to slow him down."

The laughter rippling through the group was stifled by the doctor's words, "But we're not out of the woods yet."

Words innocently spoke, unsuspectingly accepted. The path through virtually unexplored territory was chosen for them that day.

Chapter Three

Ralph's recovery was remarkable. His attitude was extremely positive, almost euphoric, at the thought of another chance at life. He knew there would be temporary limitations, but those were minor details.

Two weeks after surgery, he developed diarrhea, nausea, chills and fever and could not tolerate food. His pulse rate was irregular and his blood pressure unusually low.

Initially, the cardiovascular surgeon prescribed medication for inflammation and fluid around the heart. When Ralph's condition failed to improve, he recommended hospitalization and called in an infectious disease specialist. A series of test were ordered and it was determined that the large amounts of antibiotics given during surgery had resulted in medicine-induced colitis.

Ralph found the medication prescribed for him intolerable.

"It tastes like kerosene—my stomach is already upset—I want to go home," he said.

He was discharged a few days before Christmas.

With Ralph home and settled in bed, Bev turned her attention to Christmas preparations.

"I haven't had time to look for a Christmas tree. Would you and Jim pick one up for me?" Bev asked Rachelle, as they worked in the kitchen together.

"Mom, have you thought about an artificial tree?" Rachelle asked. "Jim and I could look for one for you if you want."

"That's not a bad idea. I might have you do that."

Ralph was roused from half-sleep by the conversation downstairs in the kitchen.

"What do they think they're doing down there," he thought, "I've been sick for two weeks and Beverly is considering buying an artificial Christmas tree without discussing it with me! An artificial Christmas tree?! Over my dead body! The next thing she'll be serving Styrofoam cookies!"

He tossed the covers back and sat up on the edge of the bed, wincing in pain from the quick movement. Weakness frustrated him. Slowly he took his robe from the end of the bed.

No one had seen Ralph walk out onto the darkened balcony in his long hooded robe.

"I have just one thing to say," he announced, raising his arm to the preaching position, his booming voice echoing off the walls, "The evergreen is symbolic of the living Christ and as long as I'm alive, there will be no artificial Christmas tree in this house!" He turned abruptly and left the balcony.

They stood gaping up at the balcony - shocked by the sight of Ralph seemingly appearing out of nowhere in his hooded robe and then disappearing almost as quickly after issuing his edict.

"For a minute there, I thought it was the Pope," Bev said in a loud whisper.

"Well," Rachelle added, a twinkle of humor in her eyes, "The 'Pope' has spoken!"

Jim laughed softly, "sounds like you're going to have a live Christmas tree. 'Chelle and I can pick one up for you tomorrow."

"Thanks, Jim, I'd appreciate it."

The next two months they focused all their attention on Ralph's recovery. Every day he and Bev walked in the shopping center, an exercise recommended by the doctors. Ralph measured his stride at home and counted his steps so he would know how far he had walked each day. By February, he was walking a mile with ease.

He returned to work late in February 1981. Although he was happy to be back in a routine, the first few days were taxing and he came home exhausted. The doctor told him it would take at least one year before he would feel good again. He waited for that time. Most of his stamina returned, but there was always a lingering tired feeling.

In the following weeks they studied nutrition. Ralph did not want to leave anything to chance. He intended to take every precaution necessary to maintain his health.

When he developed a colon inflammation a few months later, the doctors diagnosed diverticulitis and prescribed an antibiotic. The dentist prescribed an antibiotic for an infection after he had dental work done. There was still a small margin between illness and health.

Almost a year after surgery, while in North Dakota to see Laurie's new baby, Bonnie, Ralph had his first puzzling attack.

"I feel so weak and faint," Ralph said as he headed for the sofa.

Laurie put Bonnie in her infant seat near the sofa while she took his blood pressure and temperature.

"Dad, your blood pressure is 90/60, your heartbeat is irregular and you're running a low grade fever."

"Fine thing! I come up here to see my granddaughter and I have to get sick." Reaching over to touch Bonnie's chin, he said, "I wanted to take her around and show her to my friends. She has blue eyes just like mine. She even looks like me. Yes, Bonnie Lynn and I are going to get along just fine."

Bev called Ralph's cardiologist.

"What did he say?" Laurie asked.

"He said the irregular heartbeat is probably post-ventricular contractions, not indicative of anything serious. He recommended a checkup when we get back home."

"It seems it's been just one thing right after another since heart surgery," Ralph said.

Early in 1982, as a result of their nutrition studies, Ralph stopped eating refined sugar and lost 30 pounds in six weeks. His energy level also dropped, but he attributed that to low blood sugar and felt the condition would correct itself. He was delighted with his new weight as was his heart surgeon. His clothes hung on him and when he felt his weight had stabilized, he bought new clothes to fit his 5'11", 163-pound frame. He looked great!

The first breathing difficulty occurred that summer during a heat wave. Bev suggested they have an air conditioner put in, but the usual engineering style came in to play.

"If we are going to do that, it will have to be done right," Ralph said.

There would have to be a hole cut in this wall, a vent in that wall and a cold air register some place else. It became much too involved to be done before fall. The idea of an air conditioner was abandoned when the heat wave passed and the shortness of breath subsided.

"I feel so good," Ralph said one day in late September 1982. "It has taken almost two years to recover from heart surgery."

"Let's call Kathy and Steve and tell them we are coming to see our new grandson," said Bev.

Stephanie threw her arms around Ralph's leg when they arrived. "Oh, Grandpa Newman, I love you!" she said.

"I love you too, little Teffalini."

"Do you still have that black bunny rabbit in your back yard in 'Dember'?"

"Yes we do," Ralph said, "We see him almost every day."

Stephanie chattered as she led Ralph into the bedroom to show him her baby brother. "His name is Scotty," she said proudly.

"Hey, he is a good lookin' boy, and he's got blue eyes!"

Steve laughed. "I hate to disappoint you, Ralph, but his eyes are going to be brown."

"No!"

"Yeah, I'm afraid so."

"Say, Kathy, what's going on here? I thought you'd at least have one baby that looked like me."

"Sorry, Dad," she said laughing, "I'll try to do better next time."

"Okay, I'll accept that if you fix some of those fresh garden vegetables you promised me."

"You sure look great, Dad, we were pretty worried about you there for awhile."

"I feel good, Kath. It has taken a long time, but I think I have finally recovered from surgery."

Within a few days after they returned home, Ralph developed a painful inflammation of the rectum. He went through the all too familiar blood work and examinations.

"I'm not sure what is causing all of these problems I am having," Ralph said as he prepared to take his medication prescribed by the rectal specialist. "I don't think the doctors know either. I'm going to request copies of all the blood work that has been done in the past 18 months. I don't know much about medicine, but I can read."

"There is something happening with my blood," he said, after studying the test results. "There have been irregularities for eighteen months. The margin between the findings and normal has gradually increased. That tells me something is wrong, but I have no idea what. I'm thinking we should consult a hematologist. I don't like what I see here."

Laurie and Steve went to their books to try to make some sense from the information Ralph had given them. For two weeks they dug for clues. They agreed that something was not right, but there was no classic symptom pattern.

When the rectal inflammation subsided, they persuaded themselves that the problem had been resolved and they put the blood work and books away.

Chapter Four

By Thanksgiving of 1982, a vague pattern was emerging. The inflammations were becoming more frequent, and increasing in severity with each occurrence.

"I'm tired of being tired," Ralph said, as he pressed his three middle fingers to his left temple. "I should feel better than I do. It has been two years since I had surgery. I have followed all of the doctor's directions—hell—I've done more to regain my health than he recommended and I feel worse now than before I had surgery."

"Do you have that headache again?" Bev asked.

"Yes! I have this pain on the left side of my head. It always seems to come after I eat."

"You should probably get more rest," Bev said, wishing she had more to offer as a solution.

"Oh, for God's sake, Beverly! I slept for nine hours last night and got up this morning just as tired as when I went to bed. I'm trying to tell you, something isn't right. Even the guys at work have noticed it."

"What do you mean? Have they said something?"

"Yes! Dave told me today that he is scheduling me for a stress management course. I'll go along with it, but I think there is more of a problem than just stress. I don't know what it could be, though, I just got a clean bill of health from the cardiologist two weeks ago."

"Do you want to try another doctor?" Bev asked.

"I don't know, I'll see. I don't hurt any place—except for this pain on the left side of my head."

By morning, Ralph was ready for his two-mile walk. His discouragement had passed. Bev shrugged her shoulders, "Maybe Dave is right, it's probably stress," she thought.

As she waited for Ralph to come home from work that afternoon, she picked up a magazine and lazily leafed through it. She saw an article on AIDS. As she glanced through the first few paragraphs, she noted the symptoms were similar to Ralph's, but the people affected were homosexuals. As she continued to scan the article, picking up words at random, "transfusion" caught her attention. The disease could be transmitted through transfusion, but the chances were one in a million. The thought gnawed at her momentarily. "No!" she thought, "It's the 'doctor book syndrome', you read a doctor book and think you have every disease in it. The chances are only one in a million – it couldn't be. Anyway, those are vague symptoms indicative of a multitude of diseases."

Despite his reservations, Ralph enjoyed the stress management course. He hoped it was the solution to his problems. It wasn't. Three weeks into the course, he was discouraged and exhausted. The intermittent pain on the left side of this head persisted. His work schedule consumed all of his energy.

Missing R.P.'s college graduation ceremony in early December 1982 was a major disappointment.

"I sure would like to go," Ralph said, "Having a son like him is a dream come true, but I am just too tired. I hope he understands. I'm glad he's coming to work for Martin Marietta. He did a good job there last summer. I got some good reports on him. Oh, I fussed about them addressing me as R.P.'s Dad, but deep down I was proud. It will be good to have him home for a while.

Ralph chose to express his feelings in this poem he wrote in R.P.'s graduation card:

> Your college days have come and gone,
> Graduation's here, the battle's won.
> Out of the pan and into the fire,
> Keep on driving for your life's desire.
>
> Winning is easy when you have a goal,
> You've proven that by paying the toll.
> You've brought us pride and a lot of joy,
> But the apogee is, you are our boy.
>
> We can't be with upon this day,
> But our spirits will be there in every way.
> The work you have done has made us glad,
> And I'm proud to be, Just "R.P.'s Dad".

Our spirits and love will be with your forever—
Mom & Dad

Chapter Five

On Christmas Eve, 1982, the worst storm since 1913 hit Denver. Kathy, Steve and family were with Ralph and Bev for the holidays. Christmas Day came and went, but not as planned. Travel was impossible.

Rachelle's voice came over the phone too strong for the words she was saying. "Jim just ran over Jill with the van."

Fear choked any words Bev might have had in response.

"I think her leg is broken, but as far as we know she is okay otherwise. There is no ambulance service available. Jim is shoveling to get us out right now, and then we're going to take her to Aurora Community Hospital."

Ralph's emotional response to the news was inconsistent and out of character. One minute he was ranting and raving, the next minute he collapsed in a chair crying and sobbing. Despair dominated. The news had been devastating to everyone, but Ralph's reaction was a shock.

Steve and R.P. quietly left the house to shovel the driveway, while Bev tried to explain Ralph's behavior to Kathy. "Daddy hasn't been feeling well. He's just weak...that's what made him react as he did."

"What is wrong with him, Mom? We have to find out. He is so thin and pale – he looks gray," Kathy said.

With the four-wheel drive and shovels, R.P. and Steve assured them of finding a route across town to the hospital.

When they arrived at the hospital, they found Jill had sustained a broken femur, but she was doing fine.

"I'm just glad the day ended as it did and not as it might have," Ralph said.

The emotional upset and bucking of the elements was taxing and when the holidays were over, Ralph's strength had noticeably diminished.

An immobilizing chill one damp cold day in January of 1983 took its toll and Ralph came home in the middle of the afternoon.

"I just can't keep going anymore. We'll have to get to the bottom of this once and for all."

He was running a low-grade fever. They consulted the cardiologist first. His heart was checked and found to be functioning normally. A chest x-ray and blood work was ordered; the results were essentially normal, except for the irregularities in the blood work as before. The cardiologist referred them to an internist.

Ralph's weight loss, fever and shaking chills continued. There was a rash-like patch across his nose and under his eyes. The internist felt it could possibly be lupus.

Again they were all back at the books looking for answers, reading and comparing notes on everything they could find on lupus. They were distressed that treatment would be steroids, knowing the side effects of long-term use.

Bev was impatient with the doctor. "I'm going into the examining room with you. I want to know why we can't find out what's wrong."

The doctor asked, as he had before, if they had any animals in their home. They did not. "Have you been out of the country?" he asked. They had not. More tests were ordered.

"Could we possibly have the results before Friday?" Bev asked, "Because if they are negative, we can pursue another avenue before the weekend."

"I'll try," he said, not instilling the confidence she was seeking.

The fever and chills continued leaving Ralph in a state of complete exhaustion. When he was not going to the doctor or lab for tests, he slept. He slept almost 18 hours a day. His blood pressure was running 80/50 and he had lost 10 pounds in four weeks, down to 153. His new clothes began to hang as the old ones had.

He repeatedly said, "I feel like my cells are not getting enough oxygen and my legs feel as if I've been running for miles and I just got out of bed. This is the way I felt when I had double pneumonia."

The test for lupus came back negative and the doctor abandoned all thought of an autoimmune process. This was disappointing as it was the one logical lead they had. Steve and Laurie were of one mind – the problem was related to the immune system in some manner, but the pieces of the puzzle just wouldn't come together.

Every day in late afternoon, the phone would ring. "Have you found out what's wrong with Dad?" There were no answers. Bev could only express the hope that they would know more the next day. Tomorrow.

Weekends were frustrating and Mondays were like new beginnings. They were conditioned now that the answer would not be simple. They just wanted a direction.

Ralph reminded the internist of the intermittent pain on the left side of this head. Because it occurred after eating, he was convinced it was related to digestion, though there was no logical explanation for that connection.

The doctor requested a sinus series, another chest x-ray (something might have changed since the last one) and more blood work. He was bothered by the elevation of the liver enzyme, but was unsuccessful in finding a liver problem.

Another week passed, and on Friday evening the doctor called. All results were near normal or negative except the sinus x-ray, which indicated a severe sinus infection on the left side. He recommended an ear, nose and throat specialist.

Bev was totally frustrated with Ralph. Thinking he must have exaggerated his symptoms, with the end result being "nothing but a damn sinus infection."

On Monday morning, the ear, nose and throat specialist prescribed an antibiotic for 10 days.

"Would a sinus infection cause all the problems I have had?" Ralph asked.

"Oh, definitely! I have had people become deathly ill with a sinus infection," replied the doctor.

Bev was relieved that they were at last on their way out of the nightmare. She put away the thermometer, as well as the space heater she had brought into the bedroom when Ralph had been so chilled. They spoke of positive thought and how it is necessary for recovery from an illness.

The week went by with essentially no improvement, the chills and fever continued.

"I don't think we are at the root of this problem," Ralph said to Laurie during one of her late afternoon calls.

"I agree with you, Dad. There must be something else wrong. You've been on a strong dose of penicillin for 10 days and you're not getting any better. I asked a specialist here about your symptoms, and he feels there may be a tumor in the sinus cavity. Why don't you go back to the doctor again? You need more answers from him on your sinus problem."

The doctor chuckled when Ralph asked about the possibility of a tumor in the sinus cavity; it was a chuckle meant to be reassuring. He suggested that Ralph continue taking the antibiotic for another week.

"I'm also going to prescribe a six-day course of steroids, just because it will make you feel better until the medication has a chance to clear the infection."

"I'm not so sure I should be taking steroids, I don't like the side effects associated with them," Ralph said.

"A six day course won't hurt you, I take them sometimes myself just for a lift."

"That doesn't sound to me like a scientific approach," Ralph said on the way back home, "but I'll try it. If it makes me feel better, it'll be worth it."

While on the course of steroids, Ralph did feel better. His fever was gone. They concluded that even though they did not have a diagnosis, whatever was wrong would probably have to be treated with steroids. Ralph's energy and enthusiasm returned, but his color remained poor.

They enjoyed those six days, but Ralph was uneasy. "I think this is a temporary fix. I'm afraid when I finish with these tablets, I'll be back where I was before." And he was.

Whatever was wrong with Ralph was dominating their lives and taxing their patience. None of the tests had indicated a serious problem. There appeared to be no reason for Ralph's declining health. This was the thought running through Bev's mind one evening as Ralph sat at the table in his hooded robe, his head bowed, obviously despondent. She chose her words carefully.

"Ralph, I want you to search deep in your soul before you answer this question."

He looked at her, fearing her questions as much as she feared his answer.

"Are you sure you really want to get well?"

"Oh, Mom, he said, dropping his head, "Even you are beginning to wonder if this is all in my mind. I know the doctors have thought so at times. I've been concerned about that too, but why would I lose all this weight? Could my mind actually cause all these problems?"

" I don't see how it could, but I'm so confused by everything that has happened. At this point, I just wish some of the tests would be positive."

"I know what you mean, Mom......so do I."

The internist suggested seeing an infectious disease specialist.

"Would you contact him before I go in, so he knows what tests have been done?" Ralph asked the internist. "I don't want to waste time on unnecessary tests."

The doctor's office was in a huge medical center 45 minutes from home. Ralph was in the examining room less than 15 minutes.

"What did he say?" Bev asked.

Ralph's response came in a dull monotone. "He asked my symptoms and medications, he knew nothing about my case. He said 'you have been on steroids; there is nothing I can do until they are out of your system.'"

"Didn't he examine you?"

"He didn't even take my temperature!"

The drive home was quiet, neither one had anything to offer.

Slowly, methodically, Ralph built a fire in the fireplace, settled into his easy chair and sat staring into the flames.

For more than an hour he watched the fire, thoughts filtering through his mind. "I've always considered myself a rational man. I know there is something wrong with me – but if there is, why are all these doctors looking at me like I'm some sort of hypochondriac. This feeling – it's so foreign to me – I can't maintain a logical train of thought – unless I really am a mental case! Oh, God! That can't be, can it?"

He looked around the room then over at Bev. The world around him seemed otherwise normal.

"You know, he said to Bev, "Jake and Tom might be right. Maybe I should go some place else."

Chapter Six

Jake and Tom were friends from work. The three had the proper balance of personality characteristics and engineering savvy to complement each other and endure the bantering that inevitably took place when they were together.

Jake and Tom had observed the gradual decline in Ralph's health, noticing first the loss of his sense of humor, then the fatigue that plagued him. Ralph's unusual symptoms piqued their interest and challenged their analytical minds. They admitted, "We're a little out of our league," but they wanted to help find an answer.

Ralph had been hunting and cleaned rabbits and pheasants. "Could it be rabbit fever?" they asked. "The symptoms are similar, but this is by no means a classic case."

They collected information on the chemicals used in the copy room, "Could the chemical be cumulative causing some strange allergic reaction? Was he overdosing on food supplements?"

They laughed at their limited knowledge of medicine, but Ralph appreciated their concern. They too became frustrated and discouraged.

"Change your game plan...you're not getting any answers here," they said.

Ralph called the Martin Marietta doctor to get his thoughts on a course of action.

"I'm thinking about going to the Mayo Clinic," Ralph said.

The doctor's response was quick and harsh. "Stay with your doctor here, we have all the expertise you need. You just have to give them time."

After hearing a brief outline of the symptoms, he said, almost as an afterthought, "Maybe you have an adrenal dysfunction."

This provided another avenue to pursue. Within 24 hours, they had studied everything they could find on adrenal dysfunction. Steve and Laurie agreed – it was indeed a possibility.

Ralph asked the internist to test for Addison's disease, an adrenal dysfunction. His initial response was a muted snort for which he later apologized. He admitted the symptoms were similar, "But the fever doesn't fit."

"Isn't it possible that there could be two things wrong?" Ralph asked.

The doctor agreed and consented to do the necessary tests.

"A gluten intolerance can cause a lot of the symptoms you're having," Steve said.

Having nothing to lose, Bev prepared meals avoiding all use of gluten. Seeing no change in Ralph's condition after weeks, the interest in the pursuit dwindled.

Walking into the doctor's office for the adrenal function test consumed all of Ralph's energy.

"You better lie down until the doctor sees you," the nurse said.

"Thank you –I feel so tired, I guess I should."

When the test was completed, he handed the car keys to Bev. "You drive home, Mom. Just let me lie down in the back seat."

Bev was deeply concerned. For Ralph to relinquish his driving privilege was a supreme sacrifice.

The adrenal function test was negative and during one of the 5 o'clock phone conversations, Laurie told Bev of a book about urologist in New York who had coronary bypass surgery followed by similar symptoms. He had been unsuccessful in getting a diagnosis. He died and an autopsy did not provide any answers. They were fearful Ralph might be following the same course.

They spoke often of the 'guy in the book'. Bev had read it carefully for clues and found none. The book was a source of depression for Ralph.

"I don't want to hear any more about that book!" Dying is one thing, but to have all these medical people milling around not able to diagnose my problem—a man doesn't have a fighting chance of surviving if nobody knows what they're treating. Is what I have such a medical novelty that no one has ever seen it before? I might die from whatever this is, but by God, I'm going to find out what it is! If only I wasn't so tired all the time."

He reached down releasing the footrest on his red recliner, and slowly walked toward the stairs, then said to himself aloud, "I don't mind dying, but I'd at least like to know why I'm dying."

One morning he awakened feeling good. "I don't believe I have a fever. I seem to be able to breathe better. This thing may be resolving itself," he said, a sense of relief evident in his voice.

Bev was encouraged by any sign of improvement and felt a surge of energy to cope with the day, even a little excited at the thought of the black cloud leaving them.

The excitement was short-lived. Within an hour, Ralph was back in bed with the worst shaking chills he ever had. Bev put a heavy quilt on top of the bed covers and lay on top of him trying to stop his teeth-chattering chills. The shaking was so severe it brought on angina pain. With her arms around him, she cried in despair for the first time since the ordeal had begun.

The internist recommended hospitalization to allow for more sophisticated testing. The diagnosis on admission was – 'Fever of unknown origin'.

The first night in the hospital, the lab was advised to draw blood when the temperature reached 101 degrees F. For the first time in weeks, Ralph's temperature remained near normal. He was frustrated with the fish-eye he was getting from the nurses. It was midnight before his temperature began to rise and they were able to draw blood for culture.

The infectious disease specialist ordered blood work again.

"I'm beginning to wonder about you guys," Ralph said, "Are you feeding vampires? I'm not going to have any blood left."

The doctor also ordered another chest x-ray; another test for lupus and again, Ralph was asked if he had been around any animals. This time he mentioned he had been hunting in October and had cleaned rabbits and pheasants.

Because the internist still suspected a liver problem, a test was done for hepatitis. He also ordered a gallium scan.

Ralph had not heard of a gallium scan. "What is it?" he asked.

The technologist explained a radioactive isotope is injected into the vein and within 48 hours any inflamed tissue will absorb the material and thus be detected on a scan.

Bev and Rachelle watched the board carefully for scheduled tests. They queried the doctors and nurses for results. Ralph insisted on being kept informed.

When the gallium scan was completed, the x-ray technologist ordered another chest x-ray.

"Why?" Ralph asked, "I've already had four in the past two months. Can't you just look at any one of those? I understand they're all alike."

"No, Mr. Newman, with this gallium scan, your doctor will request another chest film."

"Let me see that thing!"

"I really shouldn't let you see it, you're supposed to get the results from your doctor."

"I'm here now, these are MY tests, and I want to see them."

Ralph was weak and sick, but he could still intimidate when he put his mind to it.

His lungs appeared as little tarpaper patches on the scan. The lung tissue had absorbed the radioactive isotope.

"What does this mean to you?" Ralph asked.

Shaking his head, the technologist said, "Mr. Newman, I don't know. I have never seen anything like it before."

Ralph looked again at the film, grimaced and looked back at the technologist, then back at the film.

"Even with my limited knowledge of medicine, it's obvious there is something wrong in my lungs. Isn't the reason we had this test done was to determine if any tissue would absorb the radioactive isotope?"

"Yes," the technologist responded.

"Then logically we must conclude that this is an indication of a problem in the lungs. Right?"

"Right."

"Now, all we have to do is find out what the problem is," Ralph said, turning away from the film as the technologist nodded in agreement.

Late that afternoon, Ralph walked down to the waiting room with Bev. His mood was dark, sarcasm just beneath the surface. The room was lined with people watching television, each preoccupied with their own personal crisis.

An 8-year old boy, sitting on the floor in front of the television, flipped through the channels settling on a program featuring a panel of doctors discussing terminal illnesses. As the debate progressed Ralph shifted in his chair, snuffed out his cigarette hard, the ashtray clattering on the glass tabletop, irritation evident in his action.

The T.V. host asked the panel, "What does a doctor tell his terminally ill patients?"

Sliding forward to the edge of his chair, Ralph's voice boomed through the room, "The truth! Tell them the truth! What the hell else is there?!"

His explosive statement intruded upon the passive atmosphere in the room. The momentary silence that followed ended with nervous laughter and muffled sounds of agreement. Whereupon, the startled little boy, drew back meekly volunteering, "Let's change the channel."

Chapter Seven

The next morning, Bev came to the hospital early. She wanted to hear what the doctors had to say about the test results and the gallium scan.

The two doctors entered the room at the same time followed by an assistant. The internist stood at the end of the bed by the window with his arms folded. The infectious disease specialist sat on the edge of the bed. He was a confident man, about 35 years of age, and if hazel eyes can be piercing, his were. His assistant, a slight nondescript man, stood in the background and did not speak.

Clearly, the doctor at the end of the bed was in charge. "We don't know what is wrong with you, Ralph," he said, "You are a real puzzle. You do have a sinus infection. We will be giving you an antibiotic intravenously for that. The blood culture, lupus test, hepatitis test, CAT scan and chest x-rays have all been negative."

Bev felt this was the best opportunity she would have for expression of her thoughts. "Ralph has had a lot of inflammations since surgery. Two weeks after surgery, he was readmitted with colitis. Five months later he had diverticulitis. He had a root canal done and developed an infection. He had an abscess on this rectum and in October he had a bad inflammation of his colon. I don't know how these inflammations could be related to this problem but I'm sure they are because they've all been so unusual."

They listened politely and when she was finished, they turned to each other and began talking about something else.

Ralph had found the results of the gallium scan very interesting and he was curious about their impression. "What about the gallium scan?"

"Oh, that...it was negative."

This was an occasion when Ralph's old personality flared. "If that's the case, how do you explain my lungs lighting up like a Christmas tree?"

They looked quizzically at each other then the internist nodded and quickly added, "We don't know what that means."

The doctors decided to have a private discussion in the hall. A few minutes later, the internist came back. "We've decided to do an upper G.I. series," he said.

"Guess that's the only test known to man that they haven't done," Ralph grumbled after the doctor left the room.

When the hazel-eyed doctor came in the next day, Bev asked him if he was considering looking for a common denominator to all of the inflammations since surgery.

He looked at her impatiently, with his piercing eyes and said, "What inflammations?"

"The inflammations I told you about yesterday," Bev answered.

Acting as if he had no recollection and no time to discuss it further, he snapped back, "NO!" and turned to continue a brief conversation with Ralph and left.

When the assistant stopped in that afternoon, Ralph asked him if the results of the gallium scan could indicate a severe viral pneumonia, or could this indicate damage from smoking?

The assistant ruled out both without hesitation. Coming from this young, shy man, such a confident statement was most convincing. They were again without a clue to a diagnosis.

"Do you suppose my hair dryer is emitting some carbon that has collected in my lungs?" Ralph said to Bev and Rachelle as they groped for answers.

"It's possible, Dad. At this point, we can't discount any possibility," Rachelle said.

When Bev came in the following morning, she found Ralph agitated.

"Have the doctors been in yet?" she asked, trying to determine why he was so agitated without asking.

"Yes! They've been in here. I don't know if I trust them. I don't think they know what they are doing."

Ralph had not been an easy patient to deal with. Not only did he have a problem that was difficult to diagnose, but much of the time he was impatient with hospital procedures. A great source of irritation to him was the electronic thermometers.

"Those nurses don't handle them properly. Besides that, they are not as accurate as my mercury thermometer. Bev, why don't you bring in my thermometer. They probably haven't calibrated these electronic thermometers since they were put into use. I saw a nurse drop one and then pick it up to take my temperature. You drop a piece of electronic gear like that and it's out of whack. This is just plain carelessness! Inexcusable!"

With his mercury thermometer, he took his own temperature, converted from Fahrenheit to Celsius with his calculator and told the nurses what to put on the record.

After the gallium scan incident he was determined to take charge. At the first opportunity he asked the internist to sit down for a serious talk.

"Look, the only positive data we have is the gallium scan and that revealed a problem in the lungs. Let's pursue that," Ralph said.

The doctors agreed and Ralph continued, "Now -- this is Tuesday. You guys have until Friday to come up with a diagnosis and a direction or I am leaving this hospital!"

The upper G.I. series was cancelled. A pulmonary function test revealed 1/3 normal oxygen uptake and the doctors called in a pulmonary specialist.

There was a slight awkwardness as he entered the room. He had undoubtedly been briefed on the cantankerous patient with the strange symptoms. His quiet and sincere manner was disarming. " Mr. Newman, I know this must be very difficult for you, not knowing what is causing your breathing difficulties."

"Yes it is!" I'm getting impatient with everything."

"I've studied your records and there is definitely something wrong in your lungs. We're not certain what it is, but my best guess is sarcoidosis."

"That's great! Finally we have something positive! What's sarcoidosis?"

"It's a granulomatous disorder of unknown cause. A popular theory is that exposure to pine trees could cause it."

"How do you treat it?"

"With steroids but to get a positive diagnosis, we'll have to do a bronchosopy and biopsy."

"Whatever it takes," Ralph said.

The possibility of cancer was never far from their minds, but the pulmonary specialist discounted that immediately.

Within the hour they had phoned the kids and everyone was back at their books reading what they could on sarcoidosis.

Ralph went in for a bronchoscopy with a degree of apprehension, but became interested in the procedure (performed under local anesthetic), which he was allowed to watch through a parallel scope.

When the procedure was completed, the doctor reported that he had found some definite fibrosis, but nothing unusual to indicate anything serious. "It still looks like sarcoidosis to me," he said, "but we will have to wait for the results of the biopsy to be certain."

"How long before we get the results?" Bev asked

"They should be available tomorrow and after we receive positive confirmation, we can begin treatment. Then he should be feeling good enough to return to work within one week."

That was a good day. They were happy and relieved that the whole mystery was about to end. The thought of life returning to normal was inviting.

"We may have to get an artificial Christmas tree from now on," Ralph said, "but that's a small sacrifice if I can just feel good again."

The next morning the doctors stopped by on their regular rounds. All tension was gone. They joked and laughed with Ralph.

"The people in the lab picked up on your middle name (Paul) and asked me if Paul Newman was in the hospital. I told them, 'Yes, and he is my patient.'"

Ralph and Bev did not get impatient waiting for final confirmation of the diagnosis. They were enjoying the relaxed atmosphere after weeks of upset. Rachelle and Jill came up to visit.

"Look what we brought you, Grandpa," Jill said, "A bottle of fresh-squeezed orange juice. Mom says you like that every day."

At 4 o'clock, Rachelle said, "Mom, we haven't heard from the doctors on the results of the biopsy. You better call them or we'll be sitting here waiting all weekend."

The receptionist put Bev through right away. The doctor was apologetic. "We were going to let you know – the biopsy did not indicate sarcoidosis. We're going to have to do an open-lung biopsy."

The words hit them like a thunder-ball. Ralph spoke first. "They are not going to cut me open again! We are going to the Mayo Clinic!"

Bev and Rachelle stood dumbstruck.

When Ralph's dinner tray came they decided to go down to the little Italian restaurant. They drank a half-liter of wine with their dinner, while they discussed a course of action. Bev did not look forward to calling the kids in North Dakota.

Their reaction to the latest news was predictable -- total disbelief followed by pleas to go to the Mayo Clinic.

As Bev drove back to the hospital that evening, she recalled R.P.'s words during one of their late-night conversations. As usual they were pondering a course of action. "I wonder if it's this house – maybe you should sell it. The three sixes in your 6669 house number has always bothered me," R.P. had said referencing the satanic association with those numbers.

Neither of them had taken the thought seriously. Now she was wondering – it would be a bizarre explanation for Ralph's dilemma, but thus far, they didn't have a logical one.

Ralph lay in bed after Rachelle and Bev left feeling helpless and depressed. "Here I am," he thought, "in this damn bed with no strength to fight, if or when they ever find out what I have."

When Bev returned from dinner with Rachelle, he smiled wanly. "Let's walk down to the chapel," Ralph said. He was depressed and sought peace of mind.

Ralph's attitude was one of resignation when they returned from the chapel. They spoke of what action they should take the next day. One thing they knew for certain – Ralph would be leaving the hospital the next morning.

The task of preparing to leave the hospital proved to be incredibly exhausting for Ralph. After his shower, he stood by the sink trying to breathe deeply enough to provide his body with sufficient oxygen. He rested after shaving, he rested after showering, and he rested after dressing.

Bev had not seen him in street clothes in ten days. He weighed 146 pounds, and his "new clothes" hung on him as the old ones had.

"Oh, God, I don't know if this is the right thing to do," she thought, "What if he gets home and can't get his breath? What would I do? He's talking about going to the Mayo Clinic, 1,000 miles away. How will we ever get there?"

When the internist came in, he spoke of an open-lung biopsy. Ralph was polite but firm. " I appreciate what you doctors have done. I know this is a tough problem, but I just feel I should get a second opinion. If I can't recover my health, what do I have?"

Since they had reached another blind alley, Bev asked the doctor to consider the possibility of contacting the heart center in Houston to see if any other coronary bypass patients had been found to have a similar condition. (She was thinking of the 'guy in the book').

He rejected the suggestion without time for consideration. "I don't believe there would be any advantage in that at all. I suggest you go home for the weekend, relax and consider returning for the open-lung biopsy on Monday."

"Right now I think we will be going to the Mayo Clinic," Ralph said, "Can you refer us to someone there?"

"Yes I can, if that is your decision," he said hesitantly.

Bev felt a brief pang of compassion for the doctors. They had sincerely tried to define the problem and were so disappointed at being unsuccessful. They had repeatedly rejected the suggestion of trial medication without a diagnosis, a position she respected and ultimately appreciated.

Although Ralph was convinced while in the hospital that he should go to the Mayo Clinic, once back at the coffee table in their bedroom, he was ambivalent. "What if I get so sick I can't get back home? It would be easier to have the open-lung biopsy done here. But if they still haven't found the problem, then I've removed all options."

His eyes reflected a quiet desperation as he sat slumped in the chair, his face haggard and worn. The vibrancy and zeal of 1980 was gone. It was March 1983.

Ralph's inevitable words interrupted Bev's contemplation, imposing the burden she was so reluctant to accept.

"What should we do?"

"We are going to the Mayo Clinic," she said.

Chapter Eight

Ralph looked back at the house as they left for the airport, "I wonder if I will ever see Shiloh again," he said.

At that moment Bev felt the heavy burden of her decision. She thought of the monumental error this could prove to be – then what would they do?

When they were settled in their motel that evening, the lower altitude lessened Ralph's breathing difficulties, and they were hopeful again.

The size of the Mayo Clinic building in the small Midwestern town was impressive. The walls inside were marble and cold. All the patients were classified through a priority interview. A physician took a brief history, reviewed the medical records and assigned a priority for examination. A routine classification was the lowest priority. Ralph was classified "Routine". His test findings had been essentially negative, except for the gallium scan, which was considered nonspecific.

Following the priority interview, they were directed to the east wing of the 18th floor, referred to as East 18. They couldn't know then the countless hours they would spend on East 18.

That evening Rachelle flew from Denver. Kathy, Scotty, Ralph's sister and Bev's mother arrived from North Dakota. Everyone was relieved to see Ralph less emaciated than they had imagined.

Kathy was anxious. She wanted to say the right thing. She chose the wrong words. "Gee Dad, you look good!"

Ralph had been lying in bed covered to avoid a chill. Her remark unlocked his frustrations. He worried that people were thinking he had a mental problem. He reacted by throwing back the covers, jumping out of bed an pulling off his pajama top as he spoke, "Well I don't feel very good," he said, as he revealed bony shoulders, prominent rib cage and hollow stomach. "There! Now what do you think I look like?" he said angrily.

Everyone in the room was shocked by the spontaneous action. Feeling responsible for the outburst, Kathy responded quietly, "You really are awfully thin, but I guess I was expecting you to look much worse. We all know how sick you've been."

Ralph gasped for breath from the exertion as he put his pajama top back on and crawled into bed, content that his dilemma had been properly acknowledged.

With time on their hands, they read the medical records from the Denver hospital. The history written by the hazel-eyed specialist: "This 53 year-old man was in his usual state of good health until he went hunting and cleaned rabbits and pheasants in October."

The nurse's notes implied that the patient was mentally unstable. If there were any doubts about their decision to go to the Mayo Clinic, they were dispelled.

The next morning, Ralph, and what he called his "Chinese Delegation" went back to East 18. They waited for his name to be called. At 11:30 A.M. it was. "Mr. Newman, you can go out for lunch and come back at 1:00 o'clock."

They waited from 1:00 to 4:30 for Ralph's name to be called. And it was, at 4:30 PM. He was told he could go back to the motel and come in again at 9:00 in the morning.

The next day was just like the day before. They all sat waiting with Ralph, looking at his shoes laced with the leather overlapping. He sat quietly and passively without complaint through that day and all through the next.

At the end of the third day everyone, except Ralph, was disgusted and frustrated. They spoke bitterly with an element of humor of the situation.

In desperation Bev called the doctor to whom Ralph had been referred. "I'm sorry to bother you at home doctor, but my husband is very sick. He was referred to you and has been sitting in the waiting room for three days. I believe he was classified on priority interview as a routine case. This is not a routine case. He is having so much difficulty breathing. He must have medical attention."

"Mrs. Newman, everyone who comes here and has to wait thinks they're not getting a fair shake."

"We're not so concerned that we haven't been given a fair shake as we are concerned that we have not pursued the proper course."

"You have followed the right course by starting with a priority interview," his voice softening, "Your husband will probably be seen some time tomorrow."

At 1:30 the next afternoon, Ralph walked through the entrance to the examining room, "the golden arches," as the "Chinese Delegation" referred to it.

During this preliminary examination, Doctor Morrow ordered all the tests previously done and more. The tests would be performed in rapid succession starting at 8:00 AM, Monday morning. Another frustrating weekend ahead followed by a new beginning on Monday.

Laurie and Tom arrived on Sunday with Bonnie and Jeffrey. Ralph and Bev saw their new grandson for the first time.

"He's a good lookin' boy," Ralph said, "I think he looks like me. I'm mighty proud to have him as part of my "Chinese Delegation." Jeffrey was three weeks old.

Tom casually clapped Ralph on the back, "Aw, Ralph, all your grandchildren look like you!" he said with his usual wry smile.

Ralph looked up at him and grinned; "Of course they do!" he said with mock severity, "They're all good lookin' kids!"

Tom shrugged, "What can I say?"

Ralph roared with laughter, and Tom followed suit. Ralph's laugh was always contagious.

On Monday morning, they began the trek from test to test, building to building.

Doctor Morrow met them in the subway. "I have discussed your gallium scan with some knowledgeable people, and they are not sure what it means."

As Bev watched him walk away, she said, "Oh my God! Where would one go from here?"

The next afternoon, as they waited on East 18 for Ralph's test results, Bev and the girls insisted they were going in with him. He balked but when his name was called, it was like Mother Goose and all her little goslings filing through "the golden arches".

Doctor Morrow was not surprised or intimidated by their presence. He was a confident man in his late thirties who maintained command without arrogance.

He went through the long list of test results. With minor variations they were the same as those in Denver – some irregularities but no classic pattern. The Gallium Scan again held the greatest mystery.

"There is something wrong in your lungs," Doctor Morrow quickly summarized, "but we don't know what. The only way we can diagnose your problem is with an open lung biopsy."

"Is it possible that I could have cancer?" Ralph asked.

"It is highly improbable – in fact, if this is cancer, it is the most bizarre case of cancer I've ever seen."

Doctor Morrow described the procedure and requested that Ralph be at the hospital at 7:00 that evening.

As they walked through the long corridor no one spoke. "Well, I guess I knew it would come to this," Ralph thought, "I hoped they could diagnose the problem without any more surgery, but if it has to be done, so be it. If I'm dying, I'm going to find out why!!"

When they reached the lobby, Ralph looked around at the sad faces surrounding him and said, "Somebody find a nice place for dinner. I'm taking my Chinese Delegation out to eat before I go to the hospital. It may be a while before I have a decent meal again."

The next morning the girls and Bev were in Ralph's room before he left for surgery.

"We are going to get a diagnosis today," Bev said.

"I sure hope so, Mom," sighed Ralph.

"We're going to be right here waiting for you to get out of surgery," Rachelle said, as they took turns hugging him.

"Just don't let them take me to O.R. 8," he said as the nurse wheeled him out the door.

The girls and Bev sat in the waiting room putting a jigsaw puzzle together. Two hours passed before a member of the surgical staff came in with a report. "We found nothing in the lungs to indicate malignancy. The lung tissue looks good."

"Anything from the pathologist yet?" Laurie asked.

"No, but I'll let you know as soon as I hear something."

"So far, so good, Bev said. "I'm relieved to know he doesn't have cancer," as they turned back to the distraction of their puzzle.

"Damn! There's a piece missing!" Rachelle exclaimed. "It's got to be around here someplace." The one missing puzzle piece was not to be found and was more symbolic than they realized.

Kathy was just smoothing her hand over the puzzle as the same surgical assistant hurried toward them. "We found out what it is!" he said excitedly.

Four voices in unison: "What?!" They had waited months for that moment.

"It's a parasitic pneumonia called pneumocystis carinii."

"How do you treat it?" Laurie asked.

"With an antibiotic. The IV is being put in right now."

"Thank God! At last we know – a parasitic pneumonia that can be cleared with antibiotics. I can't believe it!" Kathy exclaimed.

"A parasite! A damn parasite!" Bev said, shaking her head.

"Where did he get it?" Rachelle asked.

"We don't know," he said, "probably something he ate, I really don't know too much about it, except that nobody with a healthy immune systems gets it."

"But you can clear it with antibiotics?" Rachelle asked.

"Yes," he said weakly, slowly nodding his head. "Ah...Mr. Newman will be back in his room around 3 o'clock. You can see him then. His surgeon will be in this evening. If you have any more questions, he'll be able to answer them for you."

Bev and the girls hugged each other excitedly. Only Laurie was reserved. The reference to an unhealthy immune system troubled her.

"Let's stop by the library before we go to lunch," she said. "I've heard of pneumocystis, but I don't know much about it."

There was little to be found in the hospital library relating to the occurrence of pneumocystis in adults. Most cases dealt with congenital immunodeficiency.

"A parasite!" Bev said over lunch, "I can't believe it. This nightmare over a damn parasite."

"Dad will be so happy," Kathy said.

They were famished. They laughed over lunch and spoke of concerns they had been unwilling to voice before.

"The doctor said Dad has an unhealthy immune system, I wonder what he is talking about," Laurie said.

"We'll find out. The important thing is they can clear the problem in his lungs with antibiotics. We'll worry about the other things later," Bev said.

They couldn't wait to share the news.

"I'm going to call Jim," Rachelle said, "Brian has been so upset since Dad's been sick – this news will make him feel better."

Bev's mother had kindly consented to take care of the babies at the motel while Ralph had surgery. Bev called to share the "good news" with her. "We finally found out what's wrong with Ralph. You're not going to believe it! It's a parasite that has caused all of this!"

They were anxious to share the news with Ralph. As they hurried toward his room, their pace slowed as they caught sight of the red sticker on his door:

ISOLATION – MASKS REQUIRED

They exchanged puzzled glances, "Isolation? Why the isolation?" Kathy asked.

Laurie turned to the nurse and asked, "Do they think what he has is contagious?"

The nurse mumbled something about hospital policy and said, "The doctor will be in to see him this evening."

They put on their masks and entered the room. Ralph, groggy from the anesthetic, scarcely responded to them.

"Let's just let him rest. We'll come back this evening," Bev said.

As the approached the room that evening, they stopped, astounded to see another sticker. **GOWNS AND GLOVES REQUIRED** had been added to the isolation sticker.

"What the hell is going on?" Rachelle said, as they whirled around to find an answer.

Laurie looked down at her 3-week old son and as she saw the nurse approaching said, "Is this something contagious?" fear and bewilderment written on her face.

"I don't know if it is necessarily contagious. This is probably just a precaution since they have found another parasite."

"Another parasite?" Laurie snapped.

"Where?" Bev asked.

"You'll have to talk to the doctor when he comes. He should be here soon," the nurse replied stiffly.

They were in the room talking with Ralph when the surgeon came in. "Well, we've found out what you have," he said. "You shouldn't have it, but you do. We're giving you an antibiotic IV to clear the pneumocystis, and we'll be doing some additional testing. There is a parasite in your colon. We'll give you an antibiotic for that later."

"Is this contagious?" Bev asked, as the surgeon removed his gloves, mask and gown outside the door.

"I don't think so, but we're taking every precaution until we know more," he said, hurriedly passing through the double doors of the intensive care unit.

"I have to call Steve," Kathy said, "he should be home by now. I know he'll want to know what we've found out."

"Pneumocystis? Pneumocystis?!" Steve shouted, "That's a deadly pneumonia. Babies can be endangered by exposure to pneumocystis carinii."

When she hung up the phone, Kathy slipped into a chair, drained by Steve's reaction and the events of the day. "Steve says we shouldn't leave here until we get an answer on communicability. He is concerned about Scotty." Her words were lifeless as she leaned her head back in the chair. "It's too bad this day had to be so bittersweet."

They felt the dark clouds gathering again.

The effects of the anesthetic and the pain from the 9-inch incision in his rib cage dampened Ralph's reaction to the diagnosis. "I'm glad they finally found out what is going on in my lungs—wish they could have done it without this incision," he said, wincing as he tried to shift position, "I wonder what caused the bugs...I guess they'll let me know soon enough. At least they have found something to treat," he added with half a grin.

Apprehensively, Ralph's Chinese Delegation prepared to leave for home.

"We can't go until we have an opinion on communicability," Kathy said, "Steve will be upset if I come back home without answers to his questions."

"Oh yes, we have to have an answer to that. Also, I'm going to ask about Dad's immune system," Laurie said.

The surgeon was noncommittal on the reason for the unhealthy immune system. "We don't know yet, it could be from drugs given during heart surgery. We just have to do more testing."

As Bev left to call the hospital in Denver for the list of drugs Ralph had received, Laurie and Kathy questioned the doctor on communicability.

"... if you could please get some answers for us – these babies," Laurie said motioning to Jeffrey and Scotty, "have had close contact with Dad."

"Just let me make a couple of phone calls and I will get right back to you," the doctor replied, sensing their concern.

He returned with the words they wanted to hear. "I have consulted with all the doctors involved with this case and it is their mutual opinion that the babies are in no danger."

Although there was lingering concern, the Chinese Delegation left for home late that afternoon.

Chapter Nine

When Bev returned to the hospital that evening the "GOWN AND GLOVES" restriction had been removed from the door. Masks were required. She was surprised to see Doctor Morrow in the room as Ralph was still under the care of the surgical staff. She detected an air of tenseness; the doctor was uncomfortable and formal – not open and friendly as before.

"He thinks I might have AIDS," Ralph said, after the doctor left, "because there is something wrong with my immune system." Neither of them knew enough about AIDS to be alarmed. "If you can believe it, Doctor Morrow was asking if I had engaged in homosexual activities because of the parasites."

"Oh," Bev scoffed, mentally discounting the proposed diagnosis, "that's that homosexual disease. There is some other reason – that can't be it."

"No," Ralph chuckled, "I'm sure that's not it. The doctor was apologetic about asking the questions. I think he expected me to be upset," then shrugging, "didn't bother me. I just want to get to the bottom of this thing...speaking of that...I must let Dave know so he can notify the benefits department for me. It's nice to have a boss as a friend. Also – I have to call Jake and Tom," he laughed softly, "Those guys will be great diagnosticians someday."

After Bev left for the evening, Ralph lay motionless in his bed. He fixed his eyes on the IV in his wrist and pondered the doctor's words. "What an odd question to ask in such a serious manner," Ralph thought, "wonder what this AIDS thing is all about. Never heard of it before. Anyway it can't be what I have, because if I followed what he was saying, you get it if you're homosexual, and I am not! Why do I have this feeling that I'm in a jungle and not sure which direction to go to get out?"

The next morning, two members of the surgical staff came in on regular rounds. They were pleased with the healing of the wound, but puzzled by the pneumocystis.

"Usually we only see this in IV drug users, Haitians and......." His voice trailing off.

"And homosexuals?" Ralph said, smiling as he watched their faces.

"Yes, and homosexuals..." the doctor said, his young face flushing as he glanced at Bev.

"Mr. Newman, have you had a blood transfusion recently?"

"Just during heart surgery in 1980. That isn't very recent, but that's the only transfusion I've ever had."

Making quick mental calculation and nodding to his partner, he said, "That falls within the time frame."

Nothing more was said on the subject. They completed their examination and left.

Ralph was in the shower when Doctor Morrow came in.

"Do you have any results of the tests since surgery?" Bev asked.

"Yes, I do," he said, holding a small square of paper in the palm of his hand. Bev looked down at the hastily recorded message, but did not comprehend the gravity of his next words, "His T-cell ratio shows ten suppressor cells to one helper cell. So you see, his immune system is definitely compromised. It may return to normal after the pneumocystis clears; we will just have to wait and see."

"What can you do if it doesn't return to normal?"

"Nothing!" he said firmly.

While Bev looked at him waiting for further explanation, Ralph returned with the nurse, and the doctor directed his full attention to his patient. "Ralph, you are a real medical curiosity. All the doctors are talking about your case up and down the halls. I even walked over to the lab to check the slides myself, just to be sure the pathologist hadn't made a mistake...and the gallium scan – it is not normally used to detect pulmonary problems because it has just not proved to be effective. In this case it was invaluable."

Pleased to be part of a medical advancement, Ralph said, "Could you publish that information some place so no one else has to go through what I did to get a diagnosis?"

"I'm giving serious consideration to that. There are many curious aspects to your case. I'll let you know later on that."

Before Dr. Morrow came in the next day with Ralph's discharge orders, Bev bought a paper from the service cart to pass the time. As she casually flipped through, the italicized words, "pneumocystis carinii" leaped out at her, and she began reading to Ralph from the middle of the page, stopping after a few sentences.

Ralph had been listening intently and wondered momentarily why her voice had tapered off. He caught a glimpse of an expression on her face that worried him. "I won't press for further information now. If it is anything I need to know she'll tell me about it later," he thought, "right now all I want to do is get ready to get out of this hospital. God, how I hate hospitals!"

He smiled when the door opened and the nurse walked in. "Mr. Newman, let's get you ready to go home," she said as she helped him to his feet.

"Home." he said, "What a nice ring that word has."

When Ralph left for his shower, Bev finished reading the article. It was an entire editorial page on AIDS. The doctor had spoken of AIDS as a possible diagnosis, but it was not until then that she realized the insidiousness of the disease.

The grotesque picture at the top of the page was a skull with A-I-D-S forming the eyes, nose and mouth. The words, "There are no survivors. There is no cure," along with other information on various cases, all dead, left her totally stunned.

The newspaper rolled tightly in her hand, she moved trance-like to the door and walked woodenly out and around the circular nurses station, and back to her chair in the room. She still had the newspaper rolled in her hand when Doctor Morrow walked in.

Waving the rolled newspaper at him, she asked, "Is this what you are talking about?"

He looked at her, puzzled and confused, he couldn't possibly know what she had read.

"Are you talking about acquired immune deficiency?" she asked, carefully pronouncing each word to avoid misunderstanding.

"Oh, AIDS...yes that is what we have considered as a possible diagnosis," he said, not wishing to close the door on hope, he continued, "but, we are not positive. We'll know more when he returns on Friday."

Ralph and Bev did not speak of the diagnosis on the way to the motel. Ralph knew very little about AIDS, "And it is just as well, for now," Bev thought.

After Ralph was settled in bed and sleeping, she sat alone, thinking, "We are 1,000 miles from home, Ralph can't get out of bed alone and I'm the only one who knows what the doctor has just said. I don't want to call the kids with this – not just yet. R.P. should be here with our car sometime today. I'll talk to him first."

She was relieved to hear R.P.'s rap on the door.

Chapter Ten

R.P. enjoyed the solitude as he drove to Rochester from Denver. "Dad wants his car," he thought, "that's a sign he's feeling better. Mom and Dad will be excited to hear the news. They think Janet hung the moon – wait 'til they hear we're getting married."

He smiled with pride at having his life together. "Here I am at 22, my engineering career is off the ground, I'm buying a condominium, and I'm marrying the greatest girl in the world. I can't wait to tell Mom and Dad. These past months have been pretty rough on everybody – all that studying, searching, worrying. I'm glad it's over. Dad should be back on his feet in a month or so and everything will be back to normal - good - like it used to be."

He pulled into the motel parking lot and dashed up to the motel room, smiling broadly as he rapped on the door. He was totally unprepared for the scene awaiting him.

Bev clung to him as she said, "Oh, R.P., I'm so glad you're here. Daddy has been so sick."

"I know, Mom, but he's going to be okay now. They found out what he has and they can treat it with antibiotics...isn't that what you told me?"

"Yes, that's what I told you, but the doctors think he has AIDS."

"Wait a minute...slow down. You told me he had pneumocystis and it could be treated with antibiotics. Now what's this AIDS thing? I've never heard of it."

"I don't know much about it either, just what I read in the newspaper today," she said as she handed him the editorial page.

R.P. looked first at the picture of the skull, lifting his eyes to look at Bev, then lowering them back to the paper, shaking his head in disbelief as he read. "Where did he get it? This sounds like only homosexuals are affected."

"Read on. It says you can get it through a blood transfusion. The chances are only one in a million, but that's where the doctors think he got it."

Nothing seemed real. "One in a million? It doesn't seem possible. Are you sure?"

"No, they're not sure, more tests have been ordered. They'll let us know when we come back on Friday."

Reaching out to put his arm around his mother's shoulder, he said, "If it's true, Dad'll beat it. He's tough. We'll find some way to treat it. We've come this far, we won't let this get us down, will we?"

Ralph stirred and reached out to weakly grip R.P.'s hand. "Hi R.P., it's good to have you here."

R.P. had saved his news on his wedding plans. He wanted to share it with Mom and Dad together. "I have some good news – Janet and I are getting married in July," he said smiling smugly, waiting for their reaction. The three of them shared the first genuinely happy moment in weeks.

"I'd like to go up to Minneapolis tomorrow," Ralph said, "Colleen and Denny have been so helpful since I got sick. I'd like to visit them for a few days before I have to come back here. I need to get away from this hospital scene."

As R.P. and Bev loaded the car, Ralph sat in the chair by the small table in the motel room. He had been curious about the content of the article in the newspaper. He looked over at the dresser noticing the wrinkled newspaper peeking out from under a magazine. He pulled it over onto his lap and looked at the hideous picture of the skull. He read enough to know that he did not want to hear the doctor confirm his suspected diagnosis. "Even if he does tell me this is what I have, I can't believe there isn't something somebody somewhere can do to treat it -- and I'll find them – I'll have to find them." He tossed the paper back on the dresser and held his hand to his rib cage. Suddenly his incision was painful. "...Still feel like I'm in a jungle, and I can't tell whether I'm on my way in or on my way out," he thought as he rose to walk slowly to the door. "I hope they're ready to go. I've got to get out of here," he said softly to himself.

"You know, R.P., the doctors think I might have AIDS." Ralph said as they drove to Minneapolis. "They even asked if I was homosexual. I guess they were trying to figure out how I got it," still unaware that the disease could be contracted through blood transfusion.

"You had to get it from a transfusion, Dad...unless you have Haitian roots!" R.P. said, laughing softly.

Ralph riding in the front seat as R.P. drove snapped his head around, and pushed his heavy glasses up on his nose. "What the hell are Haitian roots?" he said gruffly, with emphasis on every word.

R.P. and Bev laughed at the unintended humor. Ralph's spirited reaction was an encouraging sign.

While in Minneapolis, Ralph enjoyed the visit with his cousin, Colleen, and Bev found the courage to call Rachelle, Laurie and Kathy to tell them the diagnosis under consideration.

Ironically, a few days before, Laurie had called Bev at the motel and said she had just heard a special on AIDS. "It sound just like what Dad has," she said.

Because there was still an element of doubt, and because they did not know much about the disease, the news had a gradual impact. Bev knew they would be digging for any information they could find.

Ralph did not improve while at Colleen's. He lost all tolerance for food, and was losing what little strength he had left.

Bev and R.P. took him back to the Mayo Clinic a day early. He accepted the help of the doorman and willingly road in a wheelchair to East 18.

Doctor Morrow greeted him warmly before he delivered the results of the recent tests. "It looks as if you do have the syndrome," he said, focusing on the records before him, not wanting to watch their faces. "We'll have to contact the Center for Disease Control. They will want to trace your blood donors since transfusion, as far as we know, was the mode of transmission."

"Right now, I'm more concerned about this nausea," Ralph said, "and look at the inside of my mouth." His mouth and tongue were coated with white yeasty patches.

"I can give you a prescription for that," Dr, Morrow said, "and I suggest that you discontinue the medication for the parasite in your colon. We'll take care of that when you feel better."

As R.P. pushed Ralph out of Dr. Morrow's office in his wheelchair, Bev turned back to the doctor and asked, "What are his chances for recovery?"

"From what we know now...ah...about 40 percent. I don't like to be too pessimistic."

"Are you saying that 60 percent of the diagnosed cases are already dead, and 40 percent are still alive?"

"Yes, that's what I'm saying."

"How long does he have?"

"About two years."

"What course does the disease take?"

"Repeated infections, each one further weakening."

"I appreciate your honesty," she said, her voice quivering as she blinked back the tears.

Dr. Morrow paused, smiling as he spoke, "One of the first things Mr. Newman told me was, 'whatever is wrong with me, tell me the truth. The only thing that will make me angry is if you don't tell me the truth.' I wish the truth had been easier to share."

Ralph sat quietly in his wheelchair as he and R.P. waited for Bev. The ugly picture of the skull flashed into his mind. He felt the inside of his mouth with his tongue as his stomach churned, amplifying his nausea and weakness. "Oh, God! I didn't want that damn diagnosis confirmed – where did this pestilence come from?" He turned to look back at R.P. and smiled wanly. The two exchanged supportive glances and squared their similar jaws – the words, "We'll fight this thing together," remained unspoken.

Chapter Eleven

When they returned to East 18 two days later, Ralph did not need a wheelchair. The intolerance for the antibiotic had caused his nausea. The medication for treatment of the pneumocystis, now taken orally, was being absorbed in adequate quantities. The chest x-ray was normal again.

The mood was much lighter in the doctor's office. He and Ralph laughed when they recalled the questioning on homosexuality.

Dr. Morrow said, "The surgeon called a conference with his assistants and me, and said, 'Okay, which one of you is going to ask this guy if he has had any homosexual relations?' He made it quite clear that he did not intend to do it. Of course, I wasn't anxious to do it either, but said I would because I'm the primary physician in your case. I didn't know what reaction I would get."

Laughing heartily, Ralph said, "I wasn't upset by your questions, I just wanted to find out what was wrong with me. I appreciate what you've done. I got some answers I didn't like, but I can't blame you for that."

"When I told the surgeon I was convinced you were telling the truth about your sexual history, he asked, 'Are you sure?' I said, this guy is no more suspect than you or I, and he didn't say any more. So we're convinced that this must have come through the blood during heart surgery."

"Thank you for your trust," Ralph said, "that's all I have to rely on."

"Our position was a difficult one also – you see, we've never seen a transfusion AIDS case here before, so we were a little skeptical."

The course of steroids remained an item of interest. The doctor spoke again of the strength, duration and dosage. "I want to be certain I have this information correct in the record. Steroids suppress the immune system – a strong dose could have killed you."

He asked Ralph to come back for a checkup in six weeks and told him to call if he had any problems in the meantime.

Although Ralph had been given a diagnosis equal to a death sentence, he refused to be discouraged. He was feeling better every day and was convinced he would regain his health.

"Let's go to North Dakota," he said to Bev, "I'm not ready to go back to Denver – besides, I want to get to know my grandchildren there." They left for North Dakota the next day.

Ralph continued to improve daily. Laurie and Kathy had been to the library and copied everything available on AIDS. "The more information we have, the better chance we have to find a treatment," Laurie said.

Ralph and Bev monitored the news constantly for any new developments. Coincidentally, there was some news on the disease almost daily. Rachelle went to the library in Denver to gather all available information. She and R.P. contacted the State Health Department in Denver and attended an AIDS forum.

They were determined to know their enemy. The battle lines had been drawn. There was no doubt—their formidable opponent was merciless and sinister beyond comprehension.

Brian was eight years old and he was confused. Grandpa Newman had answers to all his questions, but Grandpa Newman had been gone for a long time; he'd been very sick. Brian didn't ask questions; he was afraid of the answers.

After the AIDS forum, Rachelle discussed it with Jim. "I'm worried about Brian. He hasn't even mentioned Dad once since he's been gone. I know it's bothering him because he always listens when we are talking, but he won't talk about it, and he needs to get it out."

"'Chelle, this scares me – nothing can happen to Ralph; he and Brian have so much unfinished business. I don't think anyone could fill the void," Jim said, dropping his head in his hands to hide tears.

Rachelle turned and walked slowly to Brian's bedroom. She hoped she could choose the right words. "You know that Grandpa Newman has been real sick, don't you, Brian?" she said as she tucked him in.

He nodded and searched her face for some indication of what she was going to say.

"You could help Grandpa get well if you want to."

"How?" he asked, "I'd help Grandpa if I knew what to do."

"If you ask God to make him feel better, that would help him."

"Oh! Mom! That's a great idea," he said. Gleefully he hugged her, then snuggled under the covers and closed his eyes. Brian had willingly accepted induction. He was an eight-year old, small for his age, but dedicated to the cause.

A few days later, Brian came bounding up to the kitchen, "Mom! Mom! President Reagan has AIDS!"

Rachelle turned to him with an element of surprise, "What did you say?"

"I just heard on T.V. that President Reagan has AIDS!"

Jim followed Brian, chuckling, "He's talking about presidential aides," then turning to Brian, "The President has people who help him. They are called aides."

Ralph called Brian a few days later. "We're going to go out and fly those rockets we ordered as soon as I get home."

"Okay Grandpa, we're going to have fun when you get home, aren't we? Just like we used to. Right Grandpa?"

"That's right, Brian."

Chapter Twelve

At the suggestion of Dr. Morrow, Bev contacted the Center for Disease Control. They wanted to interview Ralph, and requested that she not be on the line, "....Because we have some questions of a sensitive nature to ask Mr. Newman."

Bev shrugged and dropped the receiver in the cradle. "Questions of a sensitive nature," she sniffed, looking back at the phone as Ralph continued his conversation on the extension.

"Well...what questions of a 'sensitive nature' did he ask?" she asked Ralph mockingly.

"Oh...you know...the same questions they asked at the Mayo Clinic, except he asked me if I had slept with a prostitute in the past five years."

"Well...what did you say...was that when you were groping for words? You were probably trying to decide whether it had been five or six years," she said with mock sarcasm, laughing lightly, thinking Ralph would appreciate a little humor.

Ralph was not in a mood for humor. "Bev, he said, holding his head in one hand and looking down at the table, "he said something else that I think we need to talk about."

She looked back at him as she removed his bowl of soup from the microwave. He was serious.

He motioned her to sit at the table opposite him. "Don't worry about that soup, I'm not even hungry yet."

"What's wrong?" she said as she drew her chair to the table.

"Mom, I...I'm worried where this whole thing is going. That doctor says I may have transmitted this disease to you. This is a sexually transmitted disease. He says we should avoid all sexual contact. I can handle that, but he says you could have been exposed over the past two years—after all, I've had the virus since heart surgery. Ah, Mom," he said, pushing his hair back and lifting his eyes to meet hers, "I don't want you to have to go through this...I don't want anyone to have to go through this."

He pushed his chair back from the table and walked into the living room to sit alone. "This whole thing just keeps getting worse," he thought, "I've been hoping someone will give me some good news— something!—anything that doesn't amplify the fear. I'm afraid of the scope of this goddamn thing – whatever it is, it seems I just keep getting in deeper. I do feel a little better than I did last week, though, guess I should be grateful for that."

They enjoyed the lazy days in North Dakota. The six weeks went by quickly. Ralph occupied his time by building a rabbit hutch. He had ordered black bunny rabbits for Stephanie's fourth birthday. It was good therapy for him.

A few days before their return to Rochester, he hurriedly worked on the rabbit hutch, finishing in late afternoon. Stephanie's birthday party was planned for the next day.

"There!" he said kneeling down to put the rabbits inside, "Stephanie's going to be so surprised to see you." As he smoothed their fur, a news bulletin flashed on the television: "AIDS Can Be Spread Through Routine Contact."

"Even if it isn't true, how many people will believe it now? What if it is true? Oh my God!," he said, laying his head on his arm as it rested on the rabbit hutch, "We thought we had our troubles defined—I'm afraid we've just seen the tip of the ice-burg."

Steve called that evening. He too had heard the news bulletin. "I – I don't want to hurt you Ralph, but I'm concerned about Scotty and Stephanie. I've called everybody who knows anything about AIDS and no one knows enough to assure me that a genetic weakness isn't a factor in the transmission of this disease. If it is, then Stephanie and Scotty are at risk."

"I understand your concern Steve, I wouldn't want to see those little kids hurt either," Ralph said, becoming momentarily defensive, "but we have been told by every researcher we've spoken to that AIDS can't be spread through routine contact. We're going to call the Center for Disease Control in the morning and see if we can get a straight answer."

Ralph hung up the phone and sat motionless. "Hearing that I might die in two years was bad news," he thought, "then I was told I may have transmitted this pestilence to my wife, and now this – this transmission through routine contact!! Steve is a afraid for his kids – hell, I'm afraid for his kids! I've got to get some solid information – there has to be someone who knows the facts."

Turning his chair to Bev, he said, "If Steve feels this way, and I can't really blame him, what are the people at work going to think? And what about our friends and neighbors?" Ralph was depressed; he slept very little that night.

The next morning Bev called the Center for Disease Control to ask for clarification of the bulletin.

"That is absolutely not true. AIDS cannot be spread through routine contact. We have been very upset by that erroneous report too."

Stephanie's birthday party went off as planned. Out of consideration for Steve's concerns, Ralph did not hug Stephanie and Scotty. He was content to see Stephanie surprised and excited at the sight of the black bunny rabbits.

"I'm going to name them Mr. T and Sparkly Ralph," she said.

"She was surprised, wasn't she?" Ralph asked Kathy.

"She sure was Dad," Kathy said as she threw her arms around him, crying and sobbing. "I'm so sorry, Dad, I didn't want Steve to say those things to you."

"Kathy—Kathy," he said, holding her away and looking into her eyes, "I understand Steve's fears. He's concerned about his kids. Mom and I wouldn't have it any other way. This is an ugly disease. I don't know what else to say."

Kathy called the researcher the next day for an explanation of his statement.

"I was misquoted. AIDS definitely cannot be spread through routine contact. Tell your father there is no need to refrain from hugging his grandchildren." He said, apologizing for the confusion.

Tension was relieved, but the issue had cast a shadow on Kathy and Steve's marriage that remained throughout the course of Ralph's illness.

Ralph and Bev were sad to see the "special days" end, but were anxious to get back to Rochester where another T-cell ratio would be done. From the nutrition information available, Ralph decided to take 10 grams of vitamin C daily along with ample amounts of food supplements. He also took Evening Primrose Oil, a suggestion from a biochemist. He tried it all.

They hoped there would be some improvement in the T-cell ratio, though the doctor had never encouraged them. "No one has ever recovered," he said then condescendingly adding, "but you could be the first one."

Ralph's tests were completed by early afternoon and they saw the doctor as scheduled. He recommended a thorough examination and immunologic testing for Bev, "Since this is a sexually transmitted disease, you're at risk."

They didn't realize how high their hopes were until they heard the results of Ralph's tests. The doctor had not expected any improvements in the T-cell ratio and he was right – if anything it was worse. The results of Bev's immunological testing would not be available for a few days. He would let them know by mail.

The significance of the unimproved T-cell ratio was discouraging. They were returning home with reservations. Going home always meant normal routine. Now they weren't sure what going home meant. Together, they feared the future.

Chapter Thirteen

Despite their reservations, it was good being home. Ralph's weight climbed back up to 160 pounds. His energy level improved and he returned to work in June 1983 after a four-month absence.

He was apprehensive. He wondered about his capability to handle a full schedule, and he wondered how the diagnosis would affect his relationships at work.

His concerns were unfounded. He was greeted with warmth, understanding and a degree of humor. Jake and Tom never missed a chance.

"Where do you suppose Ralph got AIDS, Tom? Jake asked.

"Gee, I don't know, Jake, the only thing we know for sure is that he isn't Haitian."

Ralph needed the work routine. He needed the bantering with Jake and Tom, and he needed life back to normal. His life was back to normal – almost.

His nightly ritual, beyond the routine, involved flushing his sinuses with salt and soda water, filling the vaporizer to keep his sinuses from drying out, swishing his mouth with medication to prevent thrush, taking his antibiotic to prevent recurrence of pneumocystis and covering his body with lotion to control skin rashes. He was religious with his evening ritual. "If this is what it takes to feel good, I'll do it," he said.

Brian enjoyed spending time with Ralph. "Grandpa and I do lots of things together, and it's fun when he feels good, but I guess he needs to rest now." Brian said to Bev as he nestled down in Ralph's red chair to watch T.V.

"Did you bring in the rest of the groceries, honey?" Bev asked.

"Yes I did, Grandma," he responded with a preoccupation that had permitted him to leave the garage door slightly ajar.

Moments later Brian called to Bev in his western drawl, peculiar to Coloradoans, "Grandma! There's a dog in the house!"

Bev looked up from her work in the kitchen to see a huge dog with pure blue eyes, looking more like an over-sized wolf than a dog! The animal paused by Ralph's red chair momentarily, turned away and walked slowly up to the kitchen. As it approached Bev jumped onto the counter as Brian ran to the bathroom and locked the door.

Bev crouched on the counter terrified. The dog, ignoring her, proceeded through into the dining room and around through the living room. Maintaining a steady pace, as if on a mission, he walked up the stairs, around the corner and into the bedroom where Ralph lay in bed with his back to the door. The dog paused by Ralph's bed to gently lick the back of his neck as if to comfort him.

At Ralph's surprised outburst, the dog turned placidly away and, maintaining his steady pace, left the house.

The mission of the blue-eyed, wolf-like dog and from whence he came, will forever remain a mystery ... he was never seen again.

The results of the tests pending when they left Rochester came from Dr. Morrow in the mail. The information was mildly encouraging. Ralph's colon parasite was no longer a significant problem. Bev's immunological tests were negative; her T-cell ratio fell within normal range.

"Thanks, God!" Ralph said to himself on hearing the news. "I couldn't have lived with myself if that test had been positive," he thought, "It's bad enough I'm in this mess, but I sure wouldn't want to feel responsible for infecting anyone else – least of all Beverly. We don't know where this ugly thing is going to lead us yet, but today I'm grateful for this news."

It was midsummer when they were in North Dakota for R.P. and Janet's wedding, that the news on Interleukin II broke. Friends and family called. They had heard there was a breakthrough on AIDS to be announced at 10 o'clock. This was the first encouraging news on AIDS. Spirits were high.

In spite of the happy stress, late hours and tight scheduling of events associated with R.P.'s wedding, Ralph did not experience a setback— a pattern so characteristic of his illness.

"I feel good. I've gained my weight back and I'm able to work full-time. From what I've read, people with AIDS are really sick...wouldn't that be something if the doctors were wrong...but I suppose that's too much to hope for," Ralph said, as he left on a business trip. He was pleased with his endurance.

R.P. was admitted to the hospital with a diagnosis of acute appendicitis on the day Ralph was scheduled to return. He went directly to the hospital, arriving 30 minutes before R.P.'s surgery.

"I know that an appendectomy is considered routine surgery," Ralph said to the nurse as she prepared to move R.P. out of the room, "but should there be a requirement for blood, it will be by designated donor."

She turned to offer reassurance, but Ralph anticipated her remarks. He threw up his hand, and said, "I don't want to hear how rare that would be – I got AIDS from a blood transfusion, and I got it here! Don't tell me about rare, just pass the word to those in attendance."

Ralph insisted on seeing R.P. in the recovery room. He refused to take the word of the nurse or doctor on R.P.'s condition.

"I'm sorry, you are not allowed to enter the recovery room, sir," the nurse said, as she stood between him and the doorway.

"I AM going to see my son!" he said, his steel blue eyes intimidating and cold, "Now, you have two choices, either you let me go in there... OR...you can bring him out here!"

"Well....why don't you go in, but just for a few minutes."

Since he had seen a television broadcast on AIDS in early May, Ralph was committed to contributing what he could to AIDS research.

There were brief flashes of bitterness. His life had changed and he was angry for himself and his family. "They don't deserve this," he thought, "and neither do I. I entered that hospital with all the faith in the world in the blood supply, and why not, in this day of advanced technology? If they didn't have control of the blood supply, then they should have disclosed that to people going in for transfusion. I could have had the option of other alternatives, like having someone I know donate blood for me. It's not just dying, but it's what I have to live with before I die – the unknowns. And God only knows what my family will be drug through before it's over."

The bitterness was generally overshadowed by his obsession for new information. The program featured AIDS patients, all homosexual, who had Kaposi's sarcoma lesions and pneumocystis. It also focused on the dangers of a contaminated blood supply. His reaction at the close of the two-part series set the tone of his attitude in the months to follow.

"I could take the pneumocystis, but I don't think I could handle that Kaposi's sarcoma. Those poor devils – I don't approve of their life style, but I have to feel sympathy for them...they're fighting to stay alive just like I am. If there is anything I can do to help find a treatment or cure, I'll do it. This disease has taught me one thing, we are our brother's keeper. I have to look at it this way...antagonism and bitterness are too taxing. I need all my strength to fight this disease."

One afternoon in September, Dr. Morrow called. "The National Institute of Health, in Baltimore, needs a transfusion AIDS patient to participate in their research program. May we submit Ralph's name?"

Bev's response came without hesitation. "Yes, he is willing to do whatever he can."

A physician from the National Institute of Health called a few days later. He explained his research program to Ralph.

"This is for evaluation purposes only. I want to make it clear that we are not offering a treatment or a cure."

"What about Interleukin II?"

"That shows more promise than anything right now, but it is not available to patients, even for experimental purposes. Once you become part of our research program, any experimental medication considered to be effective would be made available to you."

"When do I have to be there?"

"You should be here two weeks from today. We'll make all travel arrangements and let you know."

"Okay, but I'm going to the Mayo Clinic first and then to North Dakota, so I'd like to have the flight originate there instead of Denver."

"No problem. We'll be in touch."

Ralph and Bev allowed enough time for a leisurely drive to Rochester. Long distance driving was more therapeutic than tiring for Ralph. The T-cell ratio was the only measure of Ralph's immune system status and they were anxious to know what was happening. They didn't expect improvement, they only hoped it had remained stable. He was feeling good and functioning normally...they wanted him to remain so.

Dr. Morrow was surprised to see Ralph looking so healthy. On physical examination, he found no indication of new infections, and ordered the familiar series of tests. The results reporting his T-cell ratio status would be available the next afternoon.

As Dr. Morrow went through the results of the lab work, "The white cell count is within normal range...that is a very good sign." He reviewed each test result, commenting on each one, leaving the T-cell ratio until last. "There has been no improvement in the T-cell ratio. In fact, if anything it's worse." He tried to be comforting. "Please understand, this finding does not represent any significant decrease in the helper/suppressor ratio. We must allow the lab a certain latitude for error in a test such as this. You know, of course, that your immune system is severely suppressed and that has not changed."

"I know you're trying to be optimistic when you refer to laboratory error, but I have analyzed enough data in my lifetime to know that decrease, how ever small, probably is not indicative of laboratory error. Otherwise, it could easily have shown a slight increase in at least one test – but it never has, has it?" Ralph remarked flatly.

"I understand what you're saying. The only thing we can do is wait and see. As you know, there is so little known about this disease. One thing we do know is that no one has ever recovered. If the National Institute of Health has any experimental medication they feel might help you, I suggest you take it."

Although Bev's T-cell ratio fell well within normal range again, they felt no elation at hearing her findings and they were not devastated by Ralph's. A numbing process had taken place over the previous months. Nothing in the test results could surprise them.

Dr. Morrow had completed his paper on Ralph's case and gave them a copy. "It should be published in the Annals of Internal Medicine in about six weeks," he said.

Bev read the doctor's paper aloud as they drove to North Dakota.

"I hope that helps someone, at least then there would be some purpose for all this," Ralph said.

The crisp October air in North Dakota was rejuvenating. They spent four days in a positively charged atmosphere before leaving for the National Institute of Health.

"You'll be getting the latest information on AIDS straight from the 'horse's mouth'," Laurie said, as she waved goodbye.

"Get all the information you can on Interleukin II," Kathy called as they moved away, almost out of earshot.

The instructions from the National Institute of Health coordinator were very explicit. "Call transportation for a cab to the clinic. You will be interviewed for registration as an outpatient. Then you can go to your motel. Reservations have been made for you. There is a shuttle from the hotel to the clinic. The doctor will meet you at the clinic at 9:00 AM."

Chapter Fourteen

The lobby of the Clinic center was deserted except for admittance personnel, who were expecting them. "We've called the doctor to interview you," the nurse said, as she escorted them to a small glassed-in office.

Ralph was not in any discomfort, and to the casual observer, appeared to be in good health. The doctor went through the list of questions, closely watching Ralph's responses. Half way through the first page, he slowly, methodically laid his pen across the paper, lifting his head to look squarely at Ralph. He asked suspiciously, "Why are you being admitted?"

"I have AIDS."

"Oh! Excuse me!" He rose from his chair. "There is some mistake – I'm from the psychiatric department!"

Laughing lightly, Ralph said, "A few months ago I would have suspected an ulterior motive in this mistake."

The doctor left the room to speak briefly with the admittance desk. "Sorry about that," he said, when he returned, "but, since this is just a routine interview for outpatient admission, I'll just get a few more details and you can get to your motel."

A tall raw-boned doctor met them at the Clinic Center the next morning. He escorted them to the tenth floor examining room. He was courteous, but maintained a detachment from them as he explained what was known, and what was not known about AIDS. The words came easily. He outlined a schedule beginning the following morning at 8:00 AM. His Coordinator, Barbara, would be available to provide direction and answer questions. "During the course of your stay, blood will be drawn every morning, a bone marrow specimen will be taken, an eye examination will be done, and a procedure called apheresis will be done.

"Would you explain what you mean by apheresis?"

"Oh, of course," he said, "that simply means that we will draw a unit of your blood, centrifuge out the white cells, and transfuse the red cells back to you to prevent anemia."

The doctor detected nothing unusual in his examination. "You're in reasonably good shape for having a diagnosis of AIDS. What was your normal weight before you started having symptoms?"

"I weighed 180 pounds, but I dropped down to 138 pounds when I had pneumocystis."

"You weigh 160 now. That's very good. Most AIDS patients don't gain their weight back once it has been lost."

"I pay close attention to nutrition, and I take a lot of food supplements."

"Our dietitian might be interested. Anything that might help AIDS patients is of interest to us. There is still so much we don't know."

As they walked around the complex that afternoon, Bev and Ralph were overwhelmed by its size. Some of the buildings were quite old, all brick and in excellent repair. The blending of old architecture with the new was masterfully done; the grounds meticulously maintained.

As Barbara took Ralph up to the eye department, she cautioned, "You may find some of the restrictions up there objectionable."

Only his familiar grumbling enabled Bev to recognize Ralph when she returned. He was sitting in the corridor in a gown, gloves and mask; his glasses were fogged over.

"Apparently the ophthalmologist hasn't read your literature on disease transmission," Ralph said to Barbara when she came back.

She laughed, and said, "I tried to tell you."

The bone marrow specimen was taken that afternoon, with samples going to seven different departments. The apheresis was done the following afternoon.

Bev and Ralph lived in Baltimore in the mid 1950s and Ralph was feeling well enough to take a trip into the past. "Let's rent a car and drive to our old apartment."

"Okay," Bev said, "We might even find the hospital where Laurie was born. We'll get a picture of it for her. I think she'd like that."

They were pleased to see the apartment complex where they had lived was unchanged. There was a wave of nostalgia as they took pictures and reflected on the days when Rachelle and Laurie were babies.

The hospital where Laurie was born was shown on the map as a large complex. However, it was not what they expected to see. A nun passing by told them that the old St. Agnes Hospital had been torn down 20 years before. A sprawling modern brick building at the corner of a busy intersection was now St. Agnes Hospital. The stately brick building that once sat on a hill in the middle of acres of plush green lawn, castle-like in appearance, had given way to a parking lot.

"It has been 28 years since we lived here," Ralph said. "Everything changes with time."

"Yes, I know, but it's kind of disappointing," Bev said as they drove through the parking lot, onto the busy street and headed back to the motel.

The doctor summarized his findings the following day. "The fact that your white cell count falls within normal range is puzzling. All other AIDS patients we see here have half that number of white cells. With this finding, I'd be very surprised if your T-cell ratio is as bad as Mayo Clinic reports. Don't misunderstand me....the Mayo Clinic is not exactly an amateur operation," he said grinning. "That is why we are so puzzled. It will be some time before we have all the test results, but on initial evaluation, we feel you would be an excellent candidate for Interleukin. I'd suggest, since you are doing so well, that you wait until we have the genetically derived Interleukin; there will be less side effects with that."

"When do you think that will be available?" Ralph asked.

"I don't know. We have more research to do before we make the decision to do a trial. We'll let you know."

"Do you have any other suggestions for me?"

"Yes! Don't change anything. You're feeling good right now. Let's keep it that way."

He provided them with the notes recorded from the most recent AIDS conference. "When you read this, you will know what we know. Good luck now!" he said as he walked away, his long white lab coat flaring behind him. They watched him leave wishing he had more to offer yet appreciative of what he had shared.

They boarded the plane for North Dakota that afternoon. "I'm glad I had this opportunity," Ralph said. "I feel better knowing the kind of effort that is going into research."

"So do I," Bev said as they settled down to read through the AIDS conference notes.

Chapter Fifteen

They were back home in Denver when the doctor from the National Institute of Health called with more results of the tests performed. "Your T-cell ratio is the same as documented at the Mayo Clinic – severely suppressed, but we are encouraged by the favorable reaction of Interleukin with your blood. This reaffirms what we told you. You are an excellent candidate for treatment."

"Have you set up a trial on that yet?" Ralph asked.

"No, but we should have that ready in a couple of months."

About a month later, while Ralph was still basking in the good news, the call came from the Center for Disease Control. They needed a transfusion-associated AIDS patient to give blood for research. Ralph was willing, with one reservation—his blood count must be considered adequate since he had given blood at the National Institute of Health within the past month.

"Certainly, we will check that first. We will be doing an aphreresis only. You will be here for just a few hours."

"Is it possible that the apheresis could be done here and the white cells shipped?"

"No, we must have the blood fresh for this purpose."

"When do you want me there?"

"We'll make your travel arrangements for Wednesday of next week, if that won't interfere with your work schedule."

"Next Wednesday will be fine."

This was not the condition under which they had hoped to return to Atlanta, but their priorities had changed. Now they looked forward to hearing any new AIDS information.

The doctor at the National Institute of Health had briefly defined the difference in the functions of the two governmental organizations.

"We are involved in treating patients and finding a cure. The Center for Disease Control is searching to find the source of the disease, how it is transmitted and the statistics associated with it."

Ralph and Bev were interested in the theory of a Harvard scientist who suggested that a swine virus had infected pig herds in Haiti. She theorized that the people there had eaten undercooked pork, and thus contracted the disease. Coinciding with the theory was the slaughter of all pigs in Haiti in June 1983. The purpose of the mass slaughter was allegedly to prevent the spread of African swine fever to other countries in the western hemisphere.

They wanted to know if the theory had been pursued and what the results had been. They wanted to know the new statistics. They especially wanted to know if there were any documented cases of transmission from man to woman through heterosexual contact.

When they arrived in the circular drive at the CDC, they were met by the doctor's coordinator and were directed to the proper department.

The doctor shared information known about the disease. "AIDS was first acknowledged at the CDC in 1981; however, there were documented cases prior to that time. The syndrome seems to have originated in this country in New York and spread to Los Angeles and San Francisco. Now there are few states without at least one case of diagnosed AIDS. It is important that you understand what we consider to be a diagnosed case of AIDS. We do not include an immune-suppressed patient in our statistics until one of the opportunistic infections on our list is diagnosed. Until the last few months, the syndrome remained within the confines of the homosexual community. Now AIDS is creeping into the general population. We have thrown everything we can behind this program, but so far it is slow going."

"How many blood transfusion cases have been documented so far?" Ralph asked.

"There are 25 cases; about 12 of them are dead."

"How many of them are heart surgery cases?"

"I believe it is about 13."

"Have you considered the possibility that some medication given at the time of surgery could cause this immune suppression?"

"Yes, but we ruled that out because a drug-induced suppression would not last more than a few weeks."

"Do you have any documented cases of transmission from a man to a woman through sexual contact?"

"No...so far there are none that we know of. I know that is a special concern to you, and we'll surely let you know if there is anything new on that."

"How about the pigs in Haiti?"

The doctor was amused by the question. His answer was serious. "We've given that serious consideration and have not ruled out the possibility of this mode of transmission. Ralph, we are not ruling anything out until we have more facts."

When the procedure was complete, the doctor thanked Ralph and said, "Your blood will be going out as part of a panel to various research facilities. They each have a pet project and will be performing the same test on samples of blood from each risk group."

By 4 o'clock in the afternoon, they were on the flight back to Denver. A new dimension had been added to their feeling for the Old South. "I appreciate their dedication," Ralph said as he leaned back in his seat for the trip home.

A few weeks later, the Annals of Internal Medicine published Dr. Morrow's paper.

"Even though his purpose was to establish the value of the gallium scan, I appreciate this documentation in establishing my case as transfusion-related," Ralph said. "At least I won't have to worry about that issue anymore."

Ralph and Bev prepared for the holidays. Their family had grown from six to sixteen.

"This is going to be a special Christmas," Ralph said. "I want the lights strung to make those two evergreens outside look like candy canes. It will be an extra touch of class when the kids drive up, and I want music in this house throughout the holidays. This is going to be a happy time."

Ralph and Bev bought each grandchild a pair of "warm fuzzy" pajamas. The chills Ralph had endured reminded him of crawling into a cold bed when he was a child. "I don't want those little kids to ever be cold," he said.

The snow was gently falling on Christmas Eve. Ralph watched with pleasure as all his grandchildren scurried around in their new "warm fuzzy" pajamas, excited over the heaps of packages under the "live evergreen" tree.

The Christmas spirit extended through the week. When New Year's Eve came, everyone was happy to see 1983 coming to a close. It had been the most bizarre year of their lives.

It was the last day of the year. The scene was a familiar one – everyone at the kitchen table sharing thoughts and feelings.

"I should have known this year would be a bummer when I sat reading that leopard-skin coat ad and the black cat plaque fell off the fireplace," Bev said.

R.P. Laughed, "I told you I didn't like those three sixes in your address."

"Black cats, three sixes, come on..." Ralph said, "I don't believe in superstition."

"Neither do I," Kathy said, "but think of all the weird things that happened to us this year."

"Yes!" Laurie said, "remember when we arranged for all of us to go out on the houseboat when everyone was home for R.P. and Janet's wedding? We all had our nautical clothes. We were planning a fun trip – even had all the food prepared. When I made the reservations, they said 'no problem, we have two houseboats and will have one available for you.' Then the night before, a squall came up and wrecked them both. When they called to let me know, they said "this is really strange—it has never happed before.'"

"That was another one of those one-in-a-million chances," Jim said with a chuckle.

"Well, Jim, look what happened to us this year," Rachelle said, "both our cars were totaled in two separate accidents and you lost your job when Continental went chapter 11!"

"Guess it wasn't a very good year for anybody," Jim shrugged.

"Gad! For that matter, how about the next-door neighbor---come to think of it her address has three sixes too," Bev said. "You all know that Denie keeps the most immaculate house you ever laid eyes on. I couldn't believe what I saw when she called me over that afternoon last fall. Her house was full of huge black flies. They were hanging on all the windows. We killed them with magazines and scooped them up by the dustpan full. She kept saying, 'where did they come from? I don't understand this! Ask Ralph if he has any idea how this could happen – there wasn't one fly in this house when I left an hour ago!' Then when we came back from Rochester, Denie had found out that after 18 years of marriage, Dick was leaving her. It was a complete shock to her."

"Must be that 'ribbon of darkness' over me," Ralph said, feeling remotely responsible for the recounted events.

"Come on, Dad," R.P. said, "nobody can blame you for that emergency attack of appendicitis I had."

"Nor for the complications I had after Jeffrey was born," Laurie said, "As a matter of fact, I was sure glad you were there with Tom. At least they didn't transfuse me."

"They wanted to ..."Ralph said, "but Tom and I weren't about to let them do that unless it was a matter of life and death. I know this has been a tough year for all of you, but I'd like to point out that we have a lot to be grateful for - we are all here together, we're all healthy...well most of us anyway" pausing thoughtfully, "I should have known when I had that dream..."

"What dream?"

"The one about my Suburban. Back when I was recording my dreams, I had a dream that I couldn't interpret. There was a fire in my Suburban ... you all know that in dreams your car represents your body...anyway, the floor mats were burning, kind of smoldering. Some sparks flew into the back seat, but they hit the metal clasp on the seat belt and burned out. No damage was done to the back seat. I tried to put the fire out on the floor mats with tablespoons of dirty water. Eventually I got the fire out, but the floor mats were badly damaged. My interpretation of the dream is the floor mats are protective covering – like the immune system. The sparks in the back seat represent danger of transmission to my family, probably you, Mom,--you're always back-seat driving," Ralph said, as he enjoyed the interjected humor with the group. He continued with his interpretation, "the sparks did not damage the back seat, which would have to be interpreted to mean that no member of my family will be affected."

Everyone was intrigued with Ralph's dream.

"That's interesting, Ralph. Do you remember when Dr. Morrow referred to the 'smoldering' of the pneumocystis, meaning it had been abnormally slow in its progress," Bev said.

"Slow but steady," R.P. said

Ralph felt a shadow falling over the occasion. "Hey, enough of this serious talk, this is New Year's Eve. If there is any more morbid stuff, I'm canceling the party. Somebody put on some rockin' good music - - let's make the last few hours of this year light and fun."

Snacks, some champagne, and a 1,000-piece jigsaw puzzle on the dining room table (no pieces missing), and music of course. The whole family was there, a few special friends were invited, and they pushed back the furniture to dance and laugh the year away. At midnight, the strains of Auld Lang Syne reverberated off the walls as they welcomed the New Year with a champagne toast -- an unforgettable interlude.

As they crept up the stairs in the wee hours of the morning, they knew it was time to be thankful. They had family and they had love.

Chapter Sixteen

In the January 1984 issue of the New England Journal of Medicine, the Center for Disease Control published an article on transfusion-associated AIDS. Eighteen cases were included in a table; Ralph's case was one of them. Of the eighteen, studies had been completed on seven. In all of the completed studies, a member of a high-risk group was found among the donors. Ralph's case was incomplete at the time the article went to press.

The disclosure of this information prompted them to call the Center for Disease Control to inquire about blood donor tracing. The tracing of Ralph's donors was complete and a member of a high-risk group whose immune system was severely suppressed was found among them. The donor would be flown to Atlanta for evaluation.

Ralph was relieved to hear the news. "That information should remove suspicion of homosexuality from the minds of medical people who might still have reservations. Oh, I know Dr. Morrow knows better because he knows me but there are a lot of others involved who might think differently. This will be a part of my medical records now. That's good. This battle is tough enough without having to fight a silly thing like that."

Speaking of other medical personnel, "I think I should have a doctor here in Denver," Ralph said, "just in case I need immediate medical attention. Right now, I don't have anyone I can call in an emergency."

"Let's contact the National Institute of Health and ask them to recommend someone," Bev said. "They should know who is in AIDS research here."

Dr. Fraser, a soft-spoken, compassionate individual was recommended. It was he who assumed the responsibility of trudging through unknown territory with Ralph.

On initial examination he found no new infections and the blood tests paralleled previous results. Ralph was more at ease having established a rapport with a local researcher.

In mid-February the doctor from the National Institute of Health called, "Would Ralph be interested in participating in an Interleukin study? The medication would be administered intravenously five days a week for six weeks. We have some encouraging results, but permanent restoration of the immune system has not been accomplished."

"Is this the genetically derived Interleukin?" Ralph asked.

"No, we don't have that available yet. Think about it and let me know."

Ralph contacted Dr. Morrow and Dr. Fraser for their opinion - both declined comment from a medical standpoint.

"I understand your position, but what would you do if you were in my place? Forget the medical opinion!"

Their responses were similar. "If I were doing as well as you, I would probably wait for at least another six weeks. You must keep in mind, though, that the chances of experimental medication working are better if you are in reasonably good health. So this is a gamble. The final decision is yours."

Ralph and Bev had found some semblance of security in the "don't change anything" mode. They were comfortable with the decision to wait for the next trial program.

They resisted the change for a little more than six weeks, until Ralph's energy level wouldn't permit him to cope with the demands of full-time employment.

"I just need some time to rest. Then I can go back to work," he said.

Not ever returning to work was beyond comprehension for Ralph. Since he accepted the job of cleaning the photographer's studio at the age of eleven, he had always worked. It was an essential part of his life – indeed, the very fiber of his self-worth. He was at the peak of his career. He could not give up now. "It's what I've worked for all my life...I have 15 years left to enjoy it...I need the challenge....I won't let go!"

Six months later R.P. would carry three moving boxes through the front door. "Dad," he said with a heavy heart, "they had to clean out your desk today. One of the guys in your department called and asked me to pick up your things so nothing would be lost."

Ralph knew it was coming. Only a few days earlier he had received a written request to turn in his badge. He knew the corporate rules, but that didn't diminish his feeling of defeat and abandonment.

He sat at the coffee table looking at his picture on the badge, "I was a good lookin' guy then," he said to Bev with a wry smile as he handed her the badge to drop in the envelope.

"....and you still are!" she said, giving him a kiss and a long hug. She knew how much he was hurting. Holding him close, she said, "...but when you get to feeling better, you know you can always get it back," she said.

"That's right Mom, you're right," he said nodding.

"We should go to the Mayo Clinic again," Ralph said, "just to see if anything has changed. They might find an infection to treat. There has to be something wrong...I feel so bad. My T-cell count should be checked anyway."

It was the beginning of his long-term disability.

Bev had noted the increasing fatigue and loss of appetite. Of greater concern was his loss of mental alertness.

Ralph sat at the coffee table in the bedroom watching Bev pack. As she put her lavender robe in the suitcase, he said, "That's a very pretty robe, where did you get it?"

"You remember," Bev said, "you bought this for me for Christmas."

"Oh, yes, I guess I did," he responded weakly, a sick feeling in the pit of this stomach. "What's happening to my mind?" he thought, "I'm weak, tired, my mouth is full of yeast patches, and these skin rashes are driving me crazy, but my memory....what's happening to my memory? Nobody said anything about the brain being affected by this...what the hell is happening?"

The significance of the memory lapse hit Bev moments later. This was not Ralph. He spent far too much time selecting gifts and had never forgotten what he had given her.

There had been similar incidents before - puzzling incidents. No one had discussed an infection that could cause this symptom.

Their visit to the Mayo Clinic did not produce encouraging results. Ralph's T-cell ratio had decreased again. The grueling series of tests afforded no explanation for his declining health status. There was no explanation for the loss of appetite and nausea.

"This happens to all AIDS patients," Dr. Morrow said.

His words were less than comforting because translated they meant, "There is nothing we can do."

In the months to come, those words would be played back to them over and over like a haunting melody. There was nothing on the horizon for treatment. The National Institute of Health had abandoned the Interleukin program. The six-week trial had proven unsuccessful.

Ralph was at low ebb. "When Dr. Morrow said I might have to have someone help me shave, I wanted to toss in the towel right there!" Ralph said, after they returned to the motel. "I know I'm getting weaker, but there was something about hearing that I might not even have strength to shave myself that depressed me."

"Let's drive over to Milwaukee and visit the old neighborhood, Bev said, "you don't have to be back here for two days, and you've always enjoyed visiting with John."

"I don't want to visit anybody."

"But you enjoy driving."

"Yes...I do," he said hesitantly.

"Then, let's go and if you still don't want to see anyone, we'll just drive around the area where we used to live and stay in a motel."

The long drive improved Ralph's mental state. Reminiscing with John on a vibrant time in his life blotted out fear, apprehension and anger during their visit.

The AIDS epidemic was taking a far greater toll than previously predicted. The more information the researchers uncovered, the more baffling the disease became. Ralph's world was turning bleak.

Fishing was one of the few recreational activities he could enjoy. "I hear that the hours you spend fishing don't count against your life," Ralph said, his eyes tired, and only a hint of a smile.

They headed for North Dakota. The sun was setting as they drove up to Laurie and Tom's house. Bonnie bounded out of the house. "Papa Newman! Know what! The red bull killed the last unicorn!"

Ralph laughed aloud for the first time in four days.

Chapter Seventeen

During the next few days, Laurie and Bev devoted all their leisure hours to searching through medical books for a fresh approach to Ralph's problem. Somewhere in the mounds of medical information, they read of the theory that Vitamin C could strengthen the immune system. It was only a theory. Linus Pauling had been awarded the Nobel Prize for his work in Vitamin C research.

"Let's check with them," Laurie said. "They may have done some research with AIDS patients."

Bev called the Linus Pauling Institute In Washington.

"Yes, we've had some reports of anecdotal cases where AIDS patients have realized improvement in their condition after taking massive doses of Vitamin C." The doctor qualified his statement saying, "We don't have any medical history on the patients, no formal documentation." He also suggested that a trial might be worthwhile, since nothing else appeared to be working.

"Do you have any experimental programs in progress?" Bev asked.

"No, I'm sorry, we don't. We simply don't have the budget to develop a program to deal with AIDS."

"They don't have the budget, huh?" Ralph said with disgust, "Well somebody better damn well wake up and smell the coffee. Appropriation of funds shouldn't even be an issue with this rampant epidemic!"

Bev agreed, "Yes, when you think of a geometric progression, how if you take a penny and double it every day for a month you'll be a millionaire in thirty..."

"Beverly!" Ralph interrupted, "Good God, Beverly! Think! This is a hell of a lot worse than a geometric progression. The numbers have to be going up exponentially! If one person can infect 20 – think about that! It doesn't take long before you're off the charts. I don't understand where the governmental agencies are, the Department of Health and Human Services...what are they doing? And what about legislators? They remind me of Nero—fiddling while Rome burns!"

The theory from the Linus Pauling Institute was only a tiny flicker of light, but they intended to pursue it. This would be a deviation from mainstream medicine. They knew consultation on this issue with any of the doctors treating Ralph, was out of the question. They had to contact someone knowledgeable and willing to administer the treatment.

"When we get back home, I will make some calls in the Denver area," Bev said. "There has to be someone who knows what is going on in this field."

Ralph selected a quiet corner of the lake for fishing, sheltered from the cool breeze. Kathy, Stephanie and Scotty were with him. The fishing was good and the sun warmed their backs as they pretended that all was right with the world. Ralph had not had the strength and energy to develop a relationship with Scotty.

"It isn't fair to Scotty," Ralph thought, "I spent a lot of time with Brian. I know he'll remember me...and maybe Jill and Stephanie, I don't know about Bonnie, but Scotty....I don't think we've had enough time together – but at least we're going to have fun today...and we may have another chance to do this again."

"This is as a man should live," Ralph thought as he felt the sun warm his back, the summer breeze on his face, "It is the closest thing there is to peace of mind – he looked across the lake at the small clump of trees silhouetted against the horizon. He was grateful for the peaceful day. A tug on his line interrupted his meditation.

"I think I got one," he shouted as Scotty came running to his side. As the fish flipped toward shore, Scotty ran out into the lake.

"Kathy! Kathy! Catch him!" Ralph shouted.

As Kathy carried Scotty back to shore, both of them dripping wet, they laughed. They laughed together at the excitement of a little boy fishing with his grandpa.

"Grandpa—look! Grandpa—see!" Scotty cried excitedly. He had Ralph's undivided attention. The day was designed for Ralph and Scotty. It was quality time. The only time Ralph would have to truly enjoy sharing a day with Scotty. A tiny capsule of time suspended forever in memory.

When they returned to Kathy's house, Ralph was chilled and exhausted; he was running a slight fever.

Kathy was upset. The special day had been marred. "We have to do something for him," she said after Ralph was asleep. "I saw a couple on the Donahue Show a few days ago. Their little three-year-old son died of transfusion AIDS. I took their names down; they might have learned something that could help Dad. Lets' call them."

Kathy and Bev talked to the mother of the little boy. She understood their frustration, their hurt and their anger.

"It was good to talk to someone who has been through all the emotions we have," Kathy said, "but she didn't know what to do either."

"No one seems to have any answers," Bev said.

Later when Ralph awakened, Kathy and Bev related their conversation with the mother of the little boy in California.

"You mean there's someone out there who's been through this, who knows what it's like?" Ralph said, warmth showing in his eyes.

"Yes, Dad, she's been through it all," Kathy said.

"I like her already. I just wish we could sit down with her and talk. I didn't realize it before, but a support group would help a lot. I feel so alone...so isolated from the rest of the world - except my family. I don't know what I would do if I didn't have my family."

After they returned to Denver, Bev contacted an Orthomolecular specialist to ask about administration of Vitamin C intravenously, or any other suggestions he might have for Ralph.

After hearing the history of Ralph's illness, he suggested that they contact a clinic in San Diego. "They specialize in immune system therapy," he said. "If this were a member of my family, that is where I would take them."

Bev contacted the clinic in San Diego and they could give Ralph an appointment in one week.

"What've I got to lose? Let's go!" Ralph said, when Bev presented the information to him.

Because Ralph did not wish to jeopardize the relationship with Dr. Fraser, he called to tell him of his plan to go to San Diego. Dr. Fraser expressed concern that the program would create more problems than it would solve.

"I know you don't believe in this kind of treatment," Ralph said, "but it is the only game in town and I'm going to play. If it works, we've both won, if it doesn't, I'll be no worse off than I am now."

Dr. Fraser understood and wished them well. Ralph appreciated the reluctantly given blessing. He could not afford to burn any bridges.

It was June 1984. San Diego was beautiful. They were at sea level. The breeze from the ocean was warm and humid. There was a flicker of hope again.

"Maybe we should move here," Ralph said, "This hot humid air feels so good to me. I would just like to sit on the beach, dig my toes in the sand and let the sun bake me for hours. I could fish and lay on the beach in the sun. Wouldn't that be fun, Mom?"

"We can stay longer if you want to. We'd be close to the clinic, and if the program helps you – it might be the right thing to do."

"We'll think about that."

They took a cab to the motel. Ralph rested for an hour before they ventured out for a walk to the car rental office. The young man filled out the paperwork as he spoke with his girlfriend on the phone. Within 15 minutes they were off in their rental car.

The following day Ralph was examined and introduced to the regimen. "We've had some encouraging results with a few other AIDS patients, but you understand this is a very serious disease. No one has a magic bullet," the doctor said gruffly, leaning back in his chair. "All I can tell you is that we have realized successes with terminal cancer patients by working to strengthen their immune system. Of course, the major burden is on you – and you," he said nodding at Bev. "You must follow our prescribed diet. You cannot smoke, and for the first six weeks eat no red meat, fish or seafood. The only eggs you can have are those that are from closely monitored chickens."

He paused for reaction then continued, "You, Mrs. Newman, will have to learn to cook all over again. Food preparation is an important part of this program. Also you will have to give him daily injections. We offer a series of lectures and instruction classes to help you get started. Now. I suggest you take the afternoon to relax. We'll want you back here at 8:00 AM."

As they walked to their car, Ralph said, "We're going down to the harbor for lunch, and I'm going to get a different car. I don't like the way this one handles."

Neither of them chose to think or speak of the strict program.

"How are you planning to get rid of this car?" Bev asked, "We signed a six-day lease agreement."

"Oh, that's no problem. We'll just drive over to the airport and call them to come and get the car, we're leaving town! Then I'll rent one from the agency at the airport."

Ralph stepped up to the counter, confident he would have his rental car in a few minutes.

"I'm sorry, Mr. Newman, I can't rent a car to you, your driver's license is expired."

"Can we rent a car on my wife's license?"

"Of course," he said as Bev handed her license to him, "...uh...except .. Mr. Newman, your wife's license is also expired."

Turning to Bev, "How in the hell could we let this happen?" Ralph said exasperated, "Now what are we going to do?"

"You can go over the license bureau, take a test and get a temporary license," the agent volunteered, trying to be helpful.

"There's that goddamn 'ribbon of darkness' again," Ralph said sitting down in a nearby row of seat, hiking his pant leg up over his knee, scratching his leg with both hands.

"What are you doing?!" Bev asked, embarrassed.

"I don't give a damn. My leg itches and I'm frustrated – how in the hell did we let this happen?"

"God Ralph, I don't know but think about it, we've driven to Rochester, Milwaukee and North Dakota with expired licenses. When you consider it – we've really been lucky."

"Lucky, huh!" he sniffed, "Well, we can't walk to the court house. You better call a cab."

By 4 o'clock, Ralph was issued a temporary license. They drove down to the harbor. "The first rental office didn't catch the expired license. He was too busy talking to his girlfriend," Ralph said over his seafood dinner.

"If you hadn't been so fussy..."

"If I hadn't tried to get a different car, who knows how long before we'd have known about our licenses."

"See. I told you we were lucky."

They both laughed as they looked out at the sunset across the harbor.

The clinic program was rigid. It consisted of Vitamin C administered intravenously over a period of a few weeks, along with a series of daily injections, high potency vitamins orally and a strict diet that did not include meat, fish or seafood.

"No seafood!?" Ralph exclaimed. "Here I am in San Diego where I can get some of the best seafood in the world and they tell me I can't eat seafood."

"We'll start the diet after we get home," Bev said.

The program introduction included a practice session on giving injections, and instruction on food preparation. All meals had to be prepared from fresh foods. Fresh vegetables were to be scrubbed thoroughly. Any bacteria left on them would further tax the already weakened immune system.

During the four-day stay, Ralph was started on Vitamin C intravenously. It would be continued three times a week by the Orthomolecular specialist in Denver.

The time in San Diego was good for Ralph and Bev. Over the weekend, they drove 100 miles along the beach to visit Bev's sister, ate seafood down at the harbor every evening and walked to a nearby tearoom for pumpkin soup. They basked in the ocean breeze and filled their hearts with a beautiful memory.

As the plane lifted off, Bev looked down on the hazy city, small from her vantage point. She wondered if they would be permitted the opportunity of sharing another interlude such as this. They never were.

Again, they had faced the reality of going back home. Food preparation for Ralph's diet was time consuming and frustrating for Bev. Although she chose the recipes she thought Ralph would find most appealing, he was unimpressed.

"I'm sorry, but this food just doesn't appeal to me. I guess I'm not very hungry," he said, night after night – day after day. Drinking carrot juice was an important part of the diet. He couldn't tolerate it. He vomited when he tried.

"I don't think I want to move to San Diego," he said, "Much as I would like to bake in the sun and dig my toes in the sand, this program doesn't seem to be doing anything for me, and the diet stinks. I like being at home in my own bed."

After four weeks on the diet, Ralph had lost 20 pounds. He was back down to 140 pounds, weak and discouraged. He caught a glimpse of himself in the full-length mirror. "I don't even look like myself – I look like a starving old man, haggard and worn, bony and weak – what a sorry sight – reminds of the pictures of those guys in the death camps in World War II," he thought as he turned away depressed and crawled back into bed, "I'm as weak as a baby – a baby abandoned in the jungle. No one can tell me how or when I will be attacked – how long the attack will last – or if I'll wake up in the morning! Oh, they tell me I will be attacked and recover – almost – then there will be another and another and another. They can tell I will be in this jungle for at least two years and the only thing they're certain of is that I won't get out alive. 'Yup, Ralph, that's one thing we're sure of – you're not going to get out alive.' I can almost feel those damn vultures circling now."

One evening during one of Rachelle's frequent visits, she and Bev sat at the kitchen table discussing what to do.

"'Chelle, I'm tempted to take him off that diet. He's not eating, he's lost 20 pounds and we can't take the chance of more weight loss. Besides, he's miserable enough. I'd at least like to see him enjoy some of his favorite foods."

"Do you have any hamburger?" Rachelle asked.

"Yes – what are you suggesting?"

"I think we should make a macaroni casserole, wake him up and try to get him to eat. That has always been one of his favorite dishes."

As Ralph lay in bed alone, his body too tired to function, his mind too active to sleep, he thought about his family. He thought a lot about them. "How many of my grandkids will remember me? I don't want them to remember me like this – this weak, emaciated, soft-in-the-head piece of humanity. It seems like this pestilence has fragmented my brain. God! That is the one tool I need more now than ever before in my life...I feel it slipping away."

He had no physical pain but constant fatigue plagued him. His inability to think clearly, to analyze frustrated him. He was angry.

He recalled the words of the blood banking official: "Why should we be concerned about transfusion AIDS? There have only been a few cases – more people die from bee stings."

"That arrogant son-of-a bitch," Ralph thought, "he was speaking for an industry responsible for destroying my life and the lives of my family – these past months have been hard for them – and that bastard doesn't even have the decency to show any remorse! Them and their 'one-in-a-million' bullshit! ...Chances of this happening to me were one in a million? ...The rest of the story is that when it happens to you it's 100 percent!"

"We've brought you some macaroni casserole and a thick malt." Rachelle said interrupting his thoughts. Bev helped him into his long hooded robe.

"Hey, this looks good, Pooch (his pet name for Rachelle), I haven't had food like this in a long time." He ate all they served and asked for more. "Does this mean I can have hamburgers and tacos again?"

"This means you can have anything you feel like eating," Bev said. She had no intention of denying him anything he felt like eating.

Chapter Eighteen

Laurie and Kathy saw a significant change in Ralph when they came to Denver late that summer. He had not regained any weight since the 20-pound loss. His appetite remained poor even though he was permitted to eat anything he wanted. He was nauseated most of the time. His doctor in Denver recommended an examination by a gastroenterologist.

After taking a brief history of digestive problems, the gastroenterologist said, "I don't have an explanation for the nausea, except that all AIDS patients have this problem."

The frustration Bev felt at hearing those words resulted in an explosive statement. "Someone, somewhere is going to find out WHY all AIDS patients have this problem. You and I both know that an immune deficiency alone doesn't cause nausea. There has to be something wrong in his digestive tract that's causing this. We have to find it and treat it, if possible."

"We'll do an endoscopy – we might find a treatable problem."

"Bev, why don't you call Barbara at NIH. They might have some suggestions for handling this problem – could be that they have treated someone with this problem and they know what to do," Ralph said as he sat in his red chair that evening.

The next morning Bev contacted Barbara. She was concerned and understanding. "This is one of the difficulties that families are having in finding treatment for AIDS patients – some complain their doctor is requesting too many tests, others complain they aren't requesting enough. We are finding that it is necessary for every person to manage his own case. What ever you feel should, or should not be done - you must make those wishes known. I'm sorry that we don't have anything more to offer at this time. Please give Ralph our best wishes and keep in touch – I know I haven't been very helpful, but that is all I can tell you right now."

"Thanks, Barbara, we'll keep you informed. I really appreciate being able to call you when we have a question."

After she hung up she went upstairs and related the conversation to Ralph.

"Well, if that's all we've got to go on, I guess we'll have to just do the best we can with our own judgment." Ralph said, reaching his hand out, "Come and lie down with me Mom. I feel so lonesome. I need you close to me."

Within a few minutes he drifted off to sleep – a short reprieve from the turmoil.

Laurie watched Ralph for signs of a new infection. "That's a pretty productive cough you have, Dad. Has anyone done a sputum culture recently?"

"No, not since I was at the National Institute of Health nine months ago."

"We should have one done when you go in for your endoscopy on Thursday."

The results of the endoscopy were inconclusive. The doctor found white patches in the digestive tract. "I've never seen anything like it before, nor has anyone else I know. The biopsy revealed nothing. I will let you know if the sputum culture reveals anything."

In the meantime, Kathy, Laurie and Bev poured over the medical books, usually up in the bedroom. Ralph enjoyed the company. The days were warm with the bright sun shining through the window. Laurie was sitting at the table with Ralph. Kathy and Bev were sprawled on the bed, books and papers scattered around.

Ralph sat quietly, very erect, not participating in the conversation, but listening intently. His uncombed hair had noticeably thinned. One piece stood away from his head in the back. His expressionless face was haggard, pale and drawn.

Ralph was grateful for their dedication. He was frustrated and angry that he was reduced to an observer status – "but I have no choice, reading makes my head ache and it is so hard to sort out information – I can't do it – thoughts just don't come together for me," he thought as he watched the three of them search.

There was a pause in the conversation as they tried to find another piece of information to throw out for discussion. Ralph broke the silence, "Laurie – Can you help me?" he pleaded.

The three women simultaneously looked up from their books, and exchanged shocked, frightened glances.

"I'm sure going to try, Dad," Laurie said, her shoulders sagging that the thought of the responsibility.

In that brief moment, they had witnessed the passing of the baton. Their leader was staggering. The search for new information, the fight for his survival would be continued, but without his leadership.

R.P. stopped in on his way home from work. Glancing at the scene in the bedroom, he said, "Hi everybody, I see you're working on the search and destroy mission again."

"We're about ready to call for the photon torpedoes," Kathy said.

"If we just knew what we are dealing with. Is it viral or bacterial? We might have a fighting chance of coming up with the right 'weapon'," Laurie said.

"Whatever it is, it must have come from animals, because it is so foreign to the human body." Bev said.

Hours later, Laurie exclaimed, "It's a spirochete! It has to be a spirochete! I know that researchers think it's a virus, but that is a catchall for every unidentifiable medical problem. Syphilis is caused by a spirochete which was transmitted to humans from sheep. Why couldn't AIDS be caused by a spirochete transmitted to humans from the green monkey?"

"Why don't you ask the doctor about that the next time we see him?" Bev suggested.

"If we could just find out why he has no appetite – why the nausea?" Kathy said.

"When was your last stool culture done, Dad?" Laurie asked.

"I've never had one done here. I guess the last one was at the Mayo Clinic two months ago."

"How many specimens did they take at that time?"

"Just one."

"One! One? They couldn't have ruled out parasites then. Parasites in your colon could cause a lot of your symptoms. We'll ask the doctor about that too."

"I don't believe he has a parasitic infection, but I can have a stool culture done," Dr. Fraser said. "Bring the stool culture into the lab within 30 minutes from the time it is taken. We should have three separate samples over a period of five days."

The hospital laboratory was 20 miles away. Their schedule was predetermined. It was 11:30 AM when Bev and Laurie walked into the clinic center with the stool specimen. A gray-haired nurse bustled from the examining rooms.

"What is this? You mean you didn't divide the specimen into two containers?" she snapped.

"The doctor didn't tell us it had to be divided."

"I suppose I can do it, but then I'll have to take this up to the lab, and I was just on my way out for lunch," she huffed.

"Could *we* take this up the lab and have them divide it into two containers?" Bev asked.

"No! I'll do it myself, you wouldn't be able to find the lab."

Bev thought, "You rude bitch, we've been where angels fear to tread. If you can find the lab, we could probably get there blindfolded."

"Thank you," Laurie said. As they walked through the corridor Laurie added, "Mom, I always wondered what the Old Gray Mare looked like. Now I know."

The biopsy of the stomach lining came back negative. The doctor found nothing to explain the nausea. The stool culture came back negative. The only thing left was the sputum culture and so far it had shown no growth.

There had been no resolution to any of Ralph's problems. Reluctantly Kathy and Laurie prepared to leave for home.

Ralph dreaded their leaving. He needed them near him, he wanted the activity around him, they loved him and he loved them.

"I don't know what I ever did to deserve you kids, you're so good to me. This house sounds hollow already," Ralph said, "I wish this was the day you were coming, instead of the day you are leaving.

"Why don't we drive with them half way," Bev said. She knew he enjoyed driving. "We could stay in a motel and drive back home tomorrow."

Since Laurie was seven months pregnant, and Kathy two months pregnant, Steve and Tom were concerned about them driving over 700 miles through desolate territory. Ralph and Bev's decision solved more than one problem – Steve and Tom were relieved and the painful moment of saying goodbye had been delayed one more day. It was easier saying goodbye the next morning. "Call when you get home," Ralph said, as Kathy and Laurie were leaving.

Bev and Ralph were settled in at home when the phone rang.

"Mom..." Laurie hesitantly began, "Kathy is in the hospital....."

"What?!" Bev interrupted.

"Mom...Kathy and Steve left from here for home about an hour ago, but they had to come back because Kathy started hemorrhaging. She is in the hospital and they've done an ultrasound...she hasn't lost the baby, but we're concerned that she may need a transfusion."

"Has anyone donated blood for her?"

"Yes, Steve and Tom both have the same blood type. Steve has contacted the blood bank – they think we are over-reacting."

"We really don't care what they think, do we?"

"No. We don't."

"Let me know when you hear from Steve."

"Sounds like Steve is on top of the problem there," Ralph said when he heard the news, "I know he won't let them give her any blood if he doesn't know where it's coming from. I know he'll take care of her," he said through clenched teeth.

In moments of unusual stress, Ralph could not control the tightness in his jaw. He was aware of it but unable to do anything about it. He could only relax, shut out the world and go to sleep. He tried, but tossed and turned for an hour and a half before fitful sleep came to him.

Kathy was not given a transfusion. Her condition improved and she was allowed to go home a few days later. Her problem was resolved – temporarily.

Chapter Nineteen

It was July 1984. The gastroenterologist called at 7 o'clock that evening. Bev was surprised to hear from him. It had been three weeks since he had given them the results of the endoscopy and Ralph had been returned to the care of Dr. Fraser.

"May I speak to Mr. Newman?" he asked.

"This is strange," Bev thought, "They usually discuss everything with me to avoid tiring Ralph."

She handed the phone to Ralph.

"We found something!" the gastroenterologist said. "The sputum culture has shown positive for a mycobacteria. We don't know for sure what kind of mycobacteria as no one in Denver has seen it before. We will be sending it out of state for further analysis. In the meantime, we can get started on two medications and we'll add a third one when the organism is definitely identified."

Within a few minutes, Dr. Fraser called. "Ralph, I'm calling the prescription for two medications into your pharmacy. I want you to start taking them immediately."

The two doctors had something that would help Ralph. They chose to tell him the news themselves. Ralph and Bev caught a momentary glimpse of concern and compassion that went beyond the call of duty.

On one of his first visits, Ralph had told Dr. Fraser, "I'm going to make you famous. I'm going to beat this thing, with your help. Just you watch; you and I will put our heads together on this and we'll find something that works!"

As Ralph hung up the phone, he said, "I might make him famous yet."

A routine blood test revealed that Ralph was extremely anemic. He needed three units of blood. The very root of his problems was now going to be the procedure to keep him alive! A blood transfusion. Ironic.

"Yes, we want him to have the transfusion, but under no circumstances will he accept blood from the blood bank. We will select his donors," Bev told Dr. Fraser.

Dr. Fraser called the next day to tell them the blood bank had "consented" to allow Ralph to select his own donors.

They complied with all the blood bank's requirements for a "directed donation". The donors were at the blood bank well in advance of the deadline. Bev asked each donor to record the unit number, so she could be certain Ralph was given the donated blood and not a substitute unit.

At 10 o'clock on the morning of the scheduled transfusion, Dr. Fraser called. "There is only one unit available for Ralph."

"What do you mean 'available'?" Bev asked.

"R.P.'s blood has been processed and is ready for transfusion. There was only one other donor and that unit has been mistakenly sent to Boulder."

"There were two other donors," Bev said impatiently, "If I give you all of the unit numbers, do you think they can find them or will they just put a sticker on another unit of blood?"

"Oh, Mrs. Newman! That is an unnecessary fear," he responded with an element of disgust.

"I'm not afraid....just cautious," she snapped.

The unit was retrieved from Boulder and the third unit located. Ralph's transfusion was done on schedule, in spite of the blood bank's confusion.

During the transfusion, Dr. Fraser came in. "What medications are you on now?" he asked.

"You ask me that every time I see you. Are you testing my memory?" Ralph asked, half seriously, before going on to answer the question. "Ketaconozole, Isoniazid, Ethambutol, Mycostatin, Rifampin and Bactrim.....no...that's wrong. You took me off the bactrim. But shouldn't I be taking something for protection against a pneumocystis recurrence?"

"Mr. Newman, if you recall, I took you off the Bactrim when I prescribed the medication for the mycobacteria. We discussed that at the time. I felt too many medications could interact and cause more problems than they solve.

"Oh, yes, that's right, I remember now. Which reminds me of another problem I've noticed lately – my loss of short term memory."

Bev did not know until that moment that Ralph was aware of what had been nagging her for two months. She hadn't discussed her concerns with him and he had not mentioned it to her. Although they had always discussed his symptoms in detail, this was a subject that thus far had been off limits between them.

It was mid-August when Ralph and Bev consulted an attorney. He was a slender, middle-aged man, young enough to be astute and old enough to be wise. He greeted them warmly and motioned them to sit opposite his desk.

"Ralph – tell me in chronological order what happened to you," he said, with his pen poised over a yellow legal sized pad. He listened, taking notes and asking brief questions for clarification as Ralph related the events of the past 3½ years.

When Ralph was finished, he said, "I want you to know what you are getting into before we proceed with any legal action. From what you've told me, these have been hard years for both of you, but going into this kind of suit will require that you relive it again." He stopped, searching for a reaction to his ominous warning.

"Don't worry, we'll handle it," Ralph said, Bev nodding in agreement.

"Okay! I just wanted to get that out of the way. Now we have our work cut out for us. For one thing, we are taking on the largest blood center in the state, with backing from an industry with unlimited funds. We are looking at a precedent setting case involving a disease about which very little is known."

"We can prove where the blood came from, that it was contaminated, that I have AIDS and I'm going to die as a result of it," Ralph said, with only slightly veiled impatience, "What else do we need for legal action?"

The attorney paused allowing a moment to buffer emotion, then continued. "I know this has been a hell of a thing for you to endure, but unfortunately it isn't that simple. Let me just say for now, if we can get to a jury, we'll have a good chance of winning. I'll file within the next few days and then we'll get into the discovery phase which simply means pulling all the information together – then comes the tough part - finding someone in the medical profession with guts enough to testify on your behalf."

"If there's anything we can do to help, we'll do it!" Bev said, leaning forward in her chair eager for further instruction.

"How about getting a copy of the medical records from the hospital," Ralph suggested.

"That would help, especially if we can get a copy of those blood certificates," the attorney said, adding to his pages of notes.

"We'll have those for you within the week, " Ralph said looking to Bev for support.

The attorney leaned back in his padded gray chair and looked at Ralph with deep concern. "I can see that today has been a strain on you. I don't think you should come downtown again. When we meet next time, I will come to your house. That will be after I've done some homework and then I can tell you more about what will be involved in getting this case underway."

Speaking softly, he continued, "One more thing I must tell you before you leave...I don't like to say this...but if you live, this case will be worth millions. However, we know there is a chance that you won't...then the award would be significantly reduced." He raised his hand in anticipation of their next question and continued, "I know that doesn't make sense to you, but for now let me say that's just the way it works in a court of law."

"Thank you for being straight forward – above all, we have to be truthful and realistic," Ralph said reaching to shake his hand.

As they walked from the ninth floor office, Ralph linked his arm in Bev's for support.

"I feel good about him – we need him in our corner," he said weakly.

Through the congestion of downtown Denver, they slowly made their way to the parking lot.

"I'm glad we won't have to come back here again," Bev said.

It would be only a matter of months before Bev would return to the ninth floor office, her arm linked in R.P.'s for support.

The following morning, Ralph and Bev waited patiently outside the medical records office at the hospital.

"We cannot release any information without the attending physician's permission, the clerk said.

"Then I suggest you call and get his permission," Ralph responded curtly, "...and specifically, we want copies of the blood certificates."

"I'll speak to my supervisor – of course, we'll need a signed release – and how soon do you need this information?"

"I'll wait while you make the copies – I need it today."

As Ralph and Bev walked through the hospital corridor with the copies of the medical records, they were less surprised than he to meet Ralph's heart surgeon.

"Well, hello Ralph," he said, "It's good to see you. I looked for your name in the cardiology update, but I didn't see it there, I thought......"

"No one contacted me for update information," Ralph said suspiciously.

"It must have been an oversight," the doctor remarked uncomfortably.

"You know I have AIDS from the blood I received during heart surgery, don't you?" Ralph volunteered.

"Oh...do you still have that?" he said, moving toward the elevator, "you're looking good...." As the door opened he motioned farewell.

"Did you hear that?" Ralph snapped, "'Oh.... do you still have that?'" he mocked, "Wonder if he thinks I found some miracle cure."

"My God! I was given 16 units of blood!" Ralph raged, as Bev scrutinized the records, "and nobody advised me of the risks involved? Oh, I know, 'they didn't know about AIDS then,' " he sneered, "but damn it, they knew about hepatitis and other diseases in the blood. Why didn't they advise me of the risks? Why aren't they required to advise me of the risks? Is it because the blood banking industry is so uniquely secure that they don't have to cover their ass like everybody else has to do to survive? I want some answers to those questions! I deserve answers to those questions!"

A few weeks later information was released by the National Institute of Health from the Consensus Development Conference on fresh frozen plasma. The conclusion of the panel was:

"The administration of fresh frozen plasma has increased dramatically in recent years despite the paucity of definitive indications for its use. This increase has occurred in the presence of mounting evidence of its potential risks, which include viral hepatitis and possibly AIDS. Many patients who receive fresh frozen plasma can be managed more effectively and safely with alternative modalities. Appropriate use of fresh frozen plasma must be justified on clinical grounds until better evidence is available. Research to develop safer fresh frozen plasma and alternative therapies is encouraged. There is no justification for the use of fresh frozen plasma as a volume expander or as a nutritional source. Safer alternative therapies exist."

"...And I received four units of fresh frozen plasma! The virus was transmitted in one of those units of fresh frozen plasma which I didn't need!" Ralph said shaking his head despondently. "Why did they give it to me? Somebody owes me an explanation."

When the attorney arrived a few days later, he carried a brief case, which Ralph hoped contained a direction for their legal action.

"We have some very serious problems with this lawsuit," the attorney said, "Let me read you the pertinent part of the Colorado Statute, section 13-22-104(2), C.R.S. 1973, 'no physician, surgeon, hospital, blood bank, tissue bank or other person or entity who donates, obtains, prepares, transplants, injects, transfuses or otherwise transfers or who assists or participates in donating, obtaining, preparing, transplanting, injecting, transfusing or transferring any tissue, organ, blood or component thereof from one or more human beings, living or dead, for the purpose of therapy, or transplantation needed by him for his health or welfare shall be liable for any damages of any kind or description directly or indirectly caused by or resulting from any such activity; except any such person or entity remains liable for his or its own negligence or willful misconduct.' "

He placed the material in his brief case and continued, "This closes the door to everything except negligence and to establish enough evidence for that could be very difficult."

A flow of adrenalin allowed Ralph to react in a vaguely familiar way. "The constitutionality of that law should be tested!"

"Ralph, this law exists in virtually every state, it would be next to impossible to strike down."

"Okay, then what is involved in proving negligence?"

"We would have to find that the blood bank violated their standard operating procedure as approved by the Food and Drug Administration, and then find an expert witness in the medical profession with guts enough to testify."

"One of the donors of fresh frozen plasma was on unspecified medication and had a temperature of 95.7 degrees F. at the time of the donation. Does that constitute a violation of the standard operating procedure?"

"I don't know, but if that donor proves to be the same donor found to be positive for the virus, it would get us into court."

"Let's find out."

"Are you sure you want to pursue this? We're looking down the barrel of some very big guns, you know?"

Ralph sat quietly in deep thought, then snapped his head around and asked, "Did you ever hear that song about the little brown mouse?"

"No...I don't believe I have--"

"It goes....

'The liquor was spilled on the barroom floor
And the bar was closed for the night,
When out from the corner came a little brown mouse
And he danced in the pale moonlight.
He lapped up the liquor from the barroom floor
Then up on his haunches he sat
And all night long you could here him sing
Bring on the goddamn cat!'

Now as I understand that statute, this industry, in a manner of speaking, is permitted by law to fire a random bullet into the crowd and cannot be held responsible for an injured party unless the victim can prove willful misconduct. Is that right?"

"Well, Ralph, you're close," he chuckled.

"Then – Bring on the goddamn cat!"

A few days after his transfusion, Ralph was pleased to hear Bev say, "How about going to North Dakota? We can see Laurie and Tom's new baby and you can get some fishing in before the weather gets too bad up there."

"I feel better than I have in weeks. I just hope it lasts...sure...I'd like to see my new granddaughter, and I always enjoy fishing. I hope it's still nice and warm," he said, looking forward to peaceful days sitting quietly by the lake with a line in the water.

"I think I'll clean my tackle box. I don't think I've thoroughly cleaned it in 25 years."

As he sorted its contents, he reminisced as polished each lure and bobber.

"Remember when I used to take 'Chelle and Laurie fishing in Florida? The fishing was really good there, but I was young then and everything was exciting."

He rested often, finishing with his tackle box by early evening.

As he moved slowly upstairs to bed, he said, "I want to leave for North Dakota as soon as you can get things together. What did Tom and Laurie name their new baby?"

"Paula Jane."

"Did they happen to say who she looks like?"

The summer had been tiring. There had been a series of grueling tests, the severe anemia followed by the transfusions, the discovery of mycobacteria and the realization that he had short-term memory loss. Ralph and Bev looked forward to the quiet days ahead. Two days later they left to "go fishing".

Chapter Twenty

Bev called Laurie after they had settled into their motel. "We're only about 250 miles away, so we should be there by noon tomorrow."

The phone in the motel room rang at 3:30 AM. Laurie's voice was thin on the line. "I didn't want to disturb you, I know Dad needs his rest, but I thought you would want to know -- Kathy is in the hospital. She started hemorrhaging again and Steve brought her into the hospital about an hour ago. They're doing an ultrasound now. Steve will let me know as soon as he hears anything."

"What if she needs blood? Have they made any arrangements for donors?" Ralph asked as they left the motel an hour later.

This was not destined to be the peaceful retreat they had anticipated. Quite the contrary – this would be the most traumatic time they had ever spent in North Dakota, and for Ralph, the last.

After three hours of driving, Ralph became restless. Turning to Bev with a puzzled, painful grimace, he said, "Look at my hand! I can't move my fingers!" His hand was locked, the forefinger pointing down and the other three straight and rigid.

"What is wrong? You mean you can't close your hand?"

"No! It's like my fingers are frozen in this position and it's painful as hell."

"It could be that you are having some kind of spasm from gripping the wheel," Bev said, as she began to massage his hand lightly. She didn't really believe her explanation, but any other consideration was too bizarre to deal with at that time. A few minutes later, his hand relaxed and the incident passed.

As they approached the hospital, Ralph said, "I want to get some pretty red flowers for Kathy before we go up to her room."

The effects of the lower altitude were evident. Ralph was almost exuberant as he bounced into Kathy's hospital room behind a pot of red flowers.

"Hi, Kath!" he said, "What are you doing in the hospital, when I'm here to have some of those fresh garden vegetables?" The gray atmosphere in the room was momentarily lifted by his light attitude.

He wrapped his thin arms around Kathy, hugging her with all his strength. Steve's greeting was reserved. His knitted brow reflected a strain they had never seen before.

A few hours earlier, Steve had confided to Laurie that the results of the ultrasound, as interpreted at that time, were less than perfect. In fact, there was indication that the baby's head was deformed. In his discussion with Laurie, Steve had stopped short of expressing his thoughts on what might have caused it.

Laurie and Bev began their desperate search on the sly. Ralph was accustomed to the scene – books and papers scattered around. He didn't guess the purpose of the pursuit. They didn't want him to know. It would have hurt him too much.

For four days, the question haunted them. Could exposure to one of Ralph's infections, diagnosed or undiagnosed have caused a birth defect? They searched frantically for an answer.

As Ralph slept, they spoke in hushed tones, reading desperately and not liking what they found. The old cytomegalovirus (CMV) could cause very serious birth defects depending on the trimester of exposure. If the mother did not have sufficient antibodies to protect the fetus, exposure during the first trimester could cause the defect revealed in the ultrasound. Exposure during the second trimester would be less serious. Exposure during the third trimester could cause a defect not readily apparent at birth. Kathy could have been exposed in her first trimester during the July visit; Laurie in her third. They were shaken by the information they found.

Laurie and Bev now understood and shared Steve's fears. Their decision to discuss it with him was the beginning of bringing those fears into the light for closer scrutiny.

"Steve," Laurie said, "Mom and I have been doing some reading. We're concerned that some of Kathy's problems may be related to cytomegalovirus."

"Boy are you slow!" Steve replied. "I've made myself sick worrying over this thing. I know that Kathy thinks I'm just trying to be mean, but I don't want to take unnecessary risks."

"Now I'm concerned about Paula," Laurie said. "I believe we should check with the National Institute of Health to see what their position is, don't you?"

Steve agreed with the course of action, and willingly made the call.

The doctors at the National Institute of Health were noncommittal. "There are no guarantees. There is just not enough known about the disease." They gave Steve the name of the leading virologist in the United States and suggested that he call him for an opinion.

"I don't believe there is any problem with a pregnant woman being in the same room with an AIDS patient, but close contact such as hugging could be taking an unnecessary risk. If the mother does not have a sufficient antibody level for CMV, it is possible for the fetus to be adversely affected. It is not too probable, but it is possible." He suggested that a sample of Kathy's blood be submitted for testing.

117

Although Paula was only three weeks old, and appeared to be a healthy baby, prior to her birth, the doctor had noted possible intrauterine growth retardation. He had been concerned enough to order an ultrasound. Laurie worried that Paula had a birth defect that would manifest itself later.

The next day, unbeknownst to Tom, Laurie whisked Paula down to the hospital to have her blood drawn for testing. She considered it too cruel to burden Tom with her fears. He was so excited over his new baby girl.

Ralph, unaware of the drama being played out around him was too sick to attend Paula's baptism. He had another of his frequent headaches, was feverish and fatigued.

"Mom, you tell Laurie and Tom I'm sorry I couldn't make it. I hope they will understand. Wake me up when you get back and we'll have a snack while you tell me all about it."

It was early evening as Bev walked to the car. "This dreadful disease has wrapped its tentacles around the entire family," Bev thought, "and it is threatening, always threatening." The dead leaves crunched under her feet and the breeze caught her hair as the setting sun cast a long shadow, resembling a grotesque figure...a stalking ugly, unidentifiable monster. She stood with her hand on the door handle of the car staring.

"Oh God! Why has this monster been unleashed on my family? Ralph seems to understand why this is happening to him, but I don't! Please protect these innocent babies from this thing! They haven't even tasted life. Let them grow up to be strong and healthy. You won't be sorry. They will make you proud. You'll see! I know I don't have Ralph's tolerance and understanding of the way you work, but I promise I'll try to learn if you just keep that monster away from these babies!"

The "negotiation" with God left Bev with a hint of security as she drove to the baptism. It was an evening devoted to Paula Jane.

Ralph lay wide-eyed in bed after Bev left. He wanted to be a part of the special occasion. He had a new granddaughter, a new little soul

118

to add to his family, so precious, so innocent. "Thank God, she can't see all the ugly things," he thought.

The next day Kathy called from the hospital to share good news. Her regular doctor had returned from vacation and read the ultrasound. By his interpretation, there was nothing on the ultra-sound to indicate the initial bizarre findings. There was every indication that this should be a healthy baby.

"...And Mom," Kathy said, "I called the virologist. He confirmed what Steve told me. Dad can be in the same room with me without risk but close contact may present a potential problem. If Dad should happen to have an active cytomegalovirus flare-up, as AIDS patients do, it could conceivably present a threat to the baby. I feel so rotten about this, Mom, but I'm scared too!"

"I know, Kathy, we've all been scared."

"I don't want to hurt Dad, but... I.... I just don't know how to handle this, she said, crying.

"I'm going to talk to Daddy. He has to know. I'll call you later."

Bev knew she had to tell Ralph that he could not hug Kathy, and why. She chose her words carefully. "Ralph, Kathy and Steve have spoken to a very knowledgeable virologist, and he feels it would be best if you do not have close contact with Kathy, like hugging her. You may have an active CMV, which can cause birth defects. This is just a precautionary measure – just until the baby is born. Kathy was crying. She is so upset - she doesn't want to hurt you. I told her you would understand."

Ralph listened quietly, not interrupting to ask questions, nor did he immediately respond when she was finished. He sat motionless, looking out the window.

"Birth defects? Birth defects!! My God, where is this ever going to end," he thought. "If someone had opened the gates of hell and let all the evil, ugly things out, could it be worse? If that baby is affected, I can't tolerate another day on this earth! God, I ask for answers...where are the answers? God, help me."

Still staring out the window, he said, "Get Kathy on the phone."

Bev was slow to respond to his request. She didn't know what he was thinking. She didn't know what he intended to say.

"Get Kathy on the phone, please," he firmly demanded.

Bev dialed Kathy's hospital room and handed the phone to Ralph.

"Hi, Kath! What makes you think I like hugging you?" he said. They both laughed, then in a stronger voice than usual, "Not being able to hug you is a small price to pay for a healthy grandchild. Now don't be upset about this anymore! I'm a big boy now. Mom tells me you're getting out of the hospital tomorrow. That's great news!"

After he hung up the phone, the feigned enthusiasm was gone. There was a sad distant yearning in his eyes, as he recalled a time when life was good – a time before the diagnosis of AIDS had consumed their lives, a time when he was young and vibrant...fishing on the beach in Florida...'Chelle, Laurie and Kathy were so dependent, so excited over little things...planting a willow whip in the yard...he smiled faintly as he thought of how admiringly they had watched him and then announced to the whole neighborhood that they had a willow tree in their yard.

"Who would have ever thought that I would contract a homosexual disease? Now I can't even hug my own daughter!"

"This is only temporary. After the baby is born you can hug Kathy again," Bev said.

"I know, Mom, but that doesn't make today any easier." Leaning back in his chair to rest his head, he said, "Sometimes I feel as if **I** am only temporary."

Kathy and Paula's blood work revealed that neither had been exposed to the cytomegalovirus. That Kathy had no antibodies was indication that her baby had not been affected; however, to avoid possible exposure in the future was only prudent.

Ralph kept his distance from Kathy for the remainder of the vacation. His trips to his favorite fishing spot had been less frequent than he anticipated. "I always think of things I would like to do but this old body just won't cooperate."

Tom and Steve arranged to take Ralph fishing.

"I know I'm a drag for you guys but I sure do appreciate your doing this for me," Ralph said.

"Hey, we like to go fishing too," Tom said.

Laughing, Steve said, "Yeah Ralph, would you begrudge me a day off? I've been working hard you know."

"I know you have," Ralph said, "I want you guys to know how proud I am of my son-in-laws. I couldn't be happier if I had chosen my daughters' husbands myself."

"We thought you did," Tom said, as the three walked through the door laughing.

When Bev and Ralph returned early that evening, Ralph was weak and tired, but content. They had caught their limit. He never expressed a desire to go fishing again.

Ralph never spoke of dying, but on the trip back to Denver he said, "as soon as we get home, I would like to have a will drawn up. We are going to be buried in North Dakota, aren't we?"

"I suppose we probably will be," Bev said, choosing to treat it as something in the distant future.

"Back when I was a kid, I had pneumonia and the doctor said, 'There is nothing more we can do for him!' 'Dummkopf!' my grandmother scoffed after he left. She got her tea kettle full of boiling water, put a blanket over my head and sat by my bed all night long while I inhaled the steam. In a few days I was outside playing again. I'll never forget it. I wish she was here with her tea kettle now – come to think of it, I sure could go for a piece of her apple pie too. Nobody ever made apple pie like hers—yours is pretty good, Mom, but it never tasted as good as hers."

Chapter Twenty-One

Rachelle called a few days before Ralph and Bev left North Dakota. The 50 million dollar lawsuit had been filed and had received broad coverage on the local news. As a result of that publicity, an independent researcher called to ask if Ralph would participate in an experimental study. The scientists associated with the project felt they may have a medication to help AIDS patients. They wanted a transfusion AIDS patient to work with them.

"Dad, the medication hasn't been tried on humans before. I don't know if you want to get involved." Rachelle said.

"Pooch! You call them back and tell them I'm ready any time they are."

It wasn't much, but the possibility of experimental medication made the goodbyes easier, the trip home shorter.

Back home, they immediately set the wheels in motion to get started on the experimental medication. It would not be a simple task. The researchers were reluctant to release the medication without assurance that they would be credited if it worked. A Denver physician agreed to administer the program; protocols would have to be written. It would take six months for the technicalities to be resolved.

As Bev and R.P. sat on the patio enjoying the Indian summer afternoon, R.P. asked, "Mom, it seems that Dad talks with his teeth clenched more often. Do you know why he does that?"

"No, I don't, except it seems to me he does that when he is under stress."

"...And he rolls his eyes back so often and then loses his train of thought."

"I know, R.P. There is something happening with his central nervous system but nobody seems to know what."

"We've got to do something...."

"I know. I know. We're trying! Why don't you go in and see if Daddy wants to come out and have lunch with us on the patio."

R.P. walked ahead of Ralph onto the patio. As he arranged the chairs around the table, Ralph stepped onto the concrete patio and fell face down.

Bev hurried out to the patio, "What happened?" she asked kneeling down beside Ralph.

"I...I fell."

R.P. held Ralph's head as Bev slipped a pillow under him.

"Do you want us to help you back inside?" R.P. asked. "Or maybe you just want to lie on the lounge chair out here."

"Just let me get up and sit in the chair," he snapped, irritated by all the fuss and a little embarrassed by the scene.

With Ralph settled at the table, R.P. asked, "Dad what happened? Did you stub your toe on the threshold?"

"No, I didn't," Ralph responded, irritated that the subject had not been closed, "I went to step down onto the patio and it was like my leg wasn't there...I don't know why that happens."

"Happens? Did it happen before?"

"Yes, but usually it's when I get out of bed and I catch myself before I fall flat on my face."

Bev and R.P. exchanged glances.

"You just never know what's going to happen next, do you?" Ralph said, "But, you gotta' say one thing - life doesn't get dull," laughing lightly. He desperately needed to maintain some normalcy in his life. Normal to him was the father/son relationship he and R.P. had always had. It wasn't son carrying father, it was father carrying son. He didn't want that to change. He was afraid, but he didn't want R.P. -especially not R.P. - to know.

Ralph's second transfusion was scheduled for a few days before Thanksgiving. Laurie and Tom came for the holidays.

The three donors would be R.P., Jim (Rachelle's husband) and Dave, a friend of Ralph's from work.

R.P. went to the blood bank to give his blood at 7:30 AM. He carried with him the required directed donor form and completed the blood bank's questionnaire.

At 7:45 AM, R.P. called Bev. "You're not going to believe this! They said they couldn't take my blood because I've lived with an AIDS patient in the last 3 years! I tried to explain to them, but they still refused to take my blood."

"Call the doctor, he should be able to straighten this out,"

The doctor convinced the blood bank personnel that it was okay in this case to draw R.P.'s blood, inasmuch as the donated blood was being transfused to the AIDS patient with whom he had lived – his Dad.

Jim, with the necessary paper work in hand, went to donate his blood in mid-afternoon of the same day. He told the desk attendant he was there to give a directed donation for Ralph Newman.

The technologist smirked, "What is it with this guy? Is he afraid he's gonna' get AIDS?"

"No," Jim said, "he isn't afraid he's gonna' get AIDS. He's already **got** AIDS and the blood came from here."

Nothing more was said. Jim's blood was drawn and presumably processed for transfusion.

Dave donated his blood later the same day. He stated on his questionnaire that he had a skin rash and had recently been seen by a dermatologist. After consultation, it was agreed that a "hold" should be put on Dave's blood until more information could be obtained. The doctor did not wish to take the chance of transmitting any infection.

Because it was Thanksgiving weekend, it would not be possible to process another unit to replace Dave's. Ralph would receive just two units. It would take about 4 hours.

When he was admitted to the emergency room, Bev and Laurie were confident all would go smoothly. They were wrong.

As before, Bev checked the unit number and name on the first bag of blood to be certain Ralph was receiving the blood donated for him. He was receiving R.P.'s blood when his doctor walked in.

Laurie specifically wanted to ask Dr. Fraser about her spirochete theory. "I hear that the researchers believe AIDS is a virus, but the information pointing to a spirochete is most convincing. Are the researchers all in agreement that this is a virus?"

"Yes. They definitely are," he said. Then laughing softly, "Funny you should mention the spirochete idea, because that's what I thought it was too. In fact, I lost a bet to a colleague on that theory."

After the second unit of blood was in place, Bev walked over to check the unit number and name. The unit Ralph was receiving was indisputably Dave's.

"Dave's blood!? What's going on?" she exclaimed. "Damn it!! They were supposed to hold Dave's blood!"

"What?!" Laurie said in disbelief.

"This is Dave's blood! Get the nurse!"

Laurie returned with a nurse who hurriedly stopped the flow of blood into Ralph's vein.

"I'll contact the blood bank," she said, as she scurried from the room.

"Oh my God, Mom!" Laurie cried, "It's no damn wonder we're in this mess. There is no excuse for this."

When the nurse returned, she was apologetic. "I'm very sorry for this. The blood bank misunderstood the instructions and placed a hold on Jim Mollohan's blood. There will be a 45-minute delay while they process that unit. I just hope he doesn't have any reaction from this."

"I know it's not your fault. Thank you for your help," Bev said as she and the nurse walked into the corridor.

After the second unit had been transfused, the emergency room doctor spoke to R.P. as Bev helped Ralph prepare to go home. "We're very sorry for the mistake."

"Mistake! Mistake!!" R.P. lashed out. "We can't afford any more 'mistakes'. We have had three encounters with that blood bank and every one has been bungled!" Lowering his voice to regain control, he said, "I know you aren't responsible for what the blood bank did."

The incident motivated R.P. to contact politicians urging them to request tighter controls on the blood banking industry. The general response was to funnel his complaint through the Department of Health and Human Services.

The Department of Health and Human Services assured him that errors such as this were rare, but demanding directed donations increased the potential for such occurrences. This was the major reason for discouraging directed donor programs.

Chapter Twenty-Two

A few days before Thanksgiving, Jill began running a low-grade fever. She had a scratchy throat, and after three days with no improvement, Rachelle took her to the doctor. He could not explain the low-grade fever on initial examination. He suggested testing for mononucleosis.

"Jill is five years old," Bev thought. "Where would she get mono? Mono is closely related to the Epstein Barr virus and the Epstein Barr virus has been a common denominator with AIDS patients. Ralph has carried the virus since Jill was 19 months old and has had closer contact with her than any of the other grandchildren. She has always been so tiny and frail." "There are no guarantees," came echoing back from the researchers. "She had a virus six months after Ralph had surgery," Bev thought, "She was so sick and dehydrated she had to be hospitalized for IV hydration. Was that the indication of her first exposure to the AIDS virus? Ralph was hospitalized two weeks after his exposure to the virus, was dehydrated and had to have IV hydration."

There were no guarantees. The unknowns, the statements, the retractions – no one knew all the factors associated with transmission. Rachelle was aware of the unknowns as well as Bev. Each wrestled with their concerns alone.

There was relief in Rachelle's voice when she called Bev to say, "Jill's test for mono came back positive."

"Where did she get it?" Bev asked, trying to hide the anxiety she had felt for three days.

"I understand her babysitter has just recovered from mono. That must be how she was exposed."

Neither chose to reveal their deep concerns to the other. The subject was closed before it burst into further analysis.

The blood transfusions were maintaining Ralph's energy level for shorter periods of time. The weakness was gradually increasing, but something else was happening.

The regimen of daily injections, enemas, oral medication, routine monthly checkups, regularly scheduled blood transfusions and tests for new infections were more taxing than helpful to Ralph. His short-term memory loss was becoming more pronounced.

"R.P. hasn't been over for a while. I wonder what he is doing," Ralph said, as he and Bev sat at the coffee table in the bedroom.

"R.P. was over this morning before he went to work," Bev said, reminding him of the subjects discussed.

"Oh yes, I guess that's right. I seem to lose track of time," his voice trailing off.

"This will help both of us keep track of time," Bev said as she hung a calendar at the end of the dresser, a few feet away and directly opposite his chair.

The memory lapses were intermittent. Most of the time Ralph's mind was very alert. He and R.P. could discuss a technical problem in detail, he could expound at length on nutrients and how each one affects the body. He was knowledgeable of politics, and could speak intelligently on most any subject.

The memory lapses were rare, but were obvious and shocking, because they were randomly interspersed with his normally astute behavior.

"Who scribbled all over my calendar?" Ralph said agitatedly as he sat in his chair in the bedroom. "You know how it upsets me to have somebody mess up my things."

Bev whirled around to look at the calendar. Surprised and puzzled she turned slowly back to Ralph, "I...don't....see any scribbling. Do you mean this calendar?"

"Yes!! I mean that calendar!" he said angrily. "Somebody has scribbled all over it!"

"Can you read what it says?" she asked, more curious about what he was seeing than anxious over his cranky outburst.

"No! Well – it looks like there could be a big A and a big R, but mostly just scribbles, like a kid would do."

Bev took the calendar from the end of the dresser, handing it over to him. "Now show me where the scribbles are," she said gently.

He studied the calendar momentarily and slowly handed it back to Bev. "I guess there are no scribbles. I must've been seeing things," he said sheepishly.

It was a disturbing incident. It was another one of the subtle symptoms, occurring only occasionally, signifying another unidentifiable problem.

They did not discuss the incident further. Of greatest concern to Ralph was losing his mental capabilities. Bev knew that bringing this vague problem up for open discussion would have been humiliating for Ralph, and would have accomplished nothing.

"Let's go to the Food Court for tacos." She said knowing Ralph would appreciate the change of scene. There was no food he enjoyed more than tacos. They had tacos for breakfast and laughed at themselves. They considered good nutrition their business, and they were violating all the rules.

That evening the doorbell rang and Bev was surprised and pleased to see Floyd. He had been a co-worker of Ralph's, a round-faced, jolly man who laughed easily and he was concerned about Ralph. He carried with him a long slender box.

"How is Ralph doing?" he asked, discreetly laying the box on the floor.

Ralph was sitting in his red chair when Floyd walked in and shook his hand. They discussed how things were at work before Floyd brought up the long slender box.

"Ralph – I brought something that I thought you might like to try. I don't know how you feel about this sort of thing, but my mother-in-law realized some positive results during her battle with terminal cancer and I thought it might help you."

"Hey Floyd, I'm game to try anything. I haven't found anything yet that works. What is it?"

"It's a pyramid."

"A pyramid? I've studied a lot about the power of the pyramid. No one really knows why, but there is definitely something to it. Bring it in and let's try it!"

Floyd set the four aluminum poles over Ralph's red chair, aligned it with a compass and said, "Sit under this as often as you can. I'm going to check back often to see how you're doing."

After Floyd left Ralph thought more about the gesture than the effects of the pyramid. "Those guys from work, the "Swat Team", Floyd, Dave, Ed – they've walked the extra mile with me. They didn't have to. They could have been afraid of having contact with me but they never once displayed any fear. Whatever happens to me, I will never forget how considerate they have been." Ralph chuckled as he recalled his return to work after the diagnosis of AIDS. They always made light of the possibility of transmission. Joked with him about his sexual orientation to which he would respond, "Careful! Or I'll kiss you."

Over the next few weeks, Ralph did not see any significant change in his condition, but then he spent less and less time sitting in his red chair. However, the pyramid remained aligned over his chair. Ralph would not have it any other way.

Bev was unprepared when the phone rang and the voice on the other end asked to speak to "Captain Swat".

"Captain Swat?" She replied.

Ralph reached for the phone and laughed as he spoke about work and agreed to lunch at noon.

"What was that all about?" Bev asked

"Oh, didn't I tell you about the swat team"

"No."

Well Jake, Tom and Lou agreed with me some time ago that we should form a Swat Team to wipe out evil. I told them I was going to die anyway so I could be the heavy in the operation."

"...And what were you and the Swat Team going to do to eliminate evil?"

"Well, we figured we would start with Castro. I volunteered to fire the gun. Jake said he would allow me to use is shoulder to steady the gun. Of course, I told him he'd have to wear earplugs. Lou would be the strategist and Tom would run interference. We all greed that R.P. should have the honor of running up the flag."

"So today you're going to have lunch and make more plans?"

"That's right! I want you to come along though, because I'm too tired to drive both ways."

"Okay, let me help you get your clothes on and we'll go for lunch with the Swat Team." Bev said appreciating the display of spirit.

Chapter Twenty-Three

The Christmas holidays in 1984 carried only a fraction of the anticipation and excitement of the year before. Ralph was able to participate for only short periods of time.

The small family gathering on New Year's Eve lacked spirit. Where they had happily welcomed 1984, they now knew what it had held for them. Hope for Ralph's recovery had dwindled. They looked to 1985 with fear and apprehension.

The days in January were dreary. Ralph's health had noticeably deteriorated. The daily injections were discontinued. They provided no benefit for him - only discomfort. He was still faithful to his evening ritual - the mycobacteria and thrush medication along with his fiber drink in the morning.

Bev watched as he held the fiber drink to his lips. He was not drinking, just holding the glass to his lips, staring straight ahead, oblivious to anything around him. His stare was broken when his eyes rolled back revealing only the white part of his eyes. His eyes remained rolled back for a few seconds - then rolled back to their normal position. He slowly set the full glass on the table, rose from his chair and went to bed without a word.

The eyes rolling back and unusual behavior confused Bev.

"Ralph," she said shaking his shoulder gently, "What is wrong?"

He looked up staring blankly at her with pale, gray-blue eyes and then his eyelids slowly drifted shut.

She went downstairs worried, wondering.

"Now what is happening?" she said aloud, throwing her arms in the air. "What the hell is happening now?!"

She went back upstairs and tried to wake him, nudging his shoulder.

"Ralph, what is wrong, Ralph?" she asked.

He responded sleepily, "Please, just leave me alone. I'm tired."

The doctor recommended that Ralph be brought to the hospital emergency room for tests.

"Ralph, I just called the doctor," Bev said nudging him again. "He wants me to bring you to the emergency room for tests."

"No, I'm not going to the hospital. I'm staying right here in bed," he said speaking slowly and slurring his words.

Responding to his mother's plea for help, R.P. walked into the bedroom. He spoke softly. "Dad, you have to go to the hospital."

"I don't want to go to the hospital."

"You have to go – you have two choices," R.P. said, speaking gently but firmly, "One is to go willingly and the other is to be carried to the car. Which one will it be?"

R.P. wanted Ralph to see the need for medical attention. He wanted his Dad's consent. It never came.

"Mom, I'm going to have to carry him to the car."

As R.P. carried Ralph through the garage, he saw the surveying equipment meticulously stacked in the corner. He recalled his introduction to engineering. "Dad taught me how to do his drawings," he thought, "we worked together on surveying jobs. The lessons, the sharing - I was so fortunate then."

The sun reflected from the blades of the hockey skates hanging on the wall. Ralph's booming voice cheering him through a high school hockey game echoed in his mind, and the recent memory of his Dad's soft, weak words, "Why don't you use my skates? They're just like new and they're the best." He didn't want to wear his Dad's skates. He wanted his Dad to wear them and play hockey with him again.

R.P. glanced inside Ralph's big red suburban as he walked by. It had scarcely been driven these last two years. "You pick out what you think we should have for a hunting vehicle and I'll buy it," his Dad had said. He glanced through the window; the plaque was still on the dash from his Mom and Dad's vacation in 1980 – it read, "Don't hurry, don't worry and don't forget to smell the flowers."

"What flowers?" he thought bitterly. "I haven't seen any flowers lately." The duck decoys hung nearby covered with cobwebs. There had been no hunting trips these past 2 years. He felt an emptiness, a loneliness.

It was Saturday morning. As R.P. drove Ralph to the hospital, he thought how he missed the Saturday morning lectures around the kitchen table, his Dad with his cigarette and coffee, tipped back in his chair expounding on the topic of the day – drugs, drunk driving, politics, religion. "Whatever the subject, I listened and learned. Some lessons I learned better and quicker than others," R.P. thought, smiling and shaking his head as he recalled his Dad's words on the way home from the police station at 3 o'clock in the morning. His Dad never took kindly to having his Saturday morning lectures disregarded. It was 4:30 AM before his Dad finished his drinking and driving lecture ending with "and don't ever let it happen again!"

He looked over at Ralph, "I'm glad you were so strong then," he thought, "I wish you weren't so weak now."

"The doctor might find something he can treat and then you'll feel better," R.P. said hoping for a response from Ralph. Ralph sat in the seat beside R.P. staring blankly.

In the emergency room they determined that Ralph was dehydrated. He was given fluids intravenously, and became more responsive within an hour.

"Thanks R.P., I appreciate what you did. I'm sorry I acted like such a bastard, but I feel much better now. Why don't you bring Janet over when we get home. We'll order a pizza. If you'll fly, I'll buy."

"You've got yourself a deal," R.P. said reaching for his Dad's hand.

Chapter Twenty-Four

Ribaviron and Isoprinosene were widely rumored to be helpful in treating AIDS. Ralph and Bev sought out all available information. It was not approved by the FDA for sale in the United States but was available across the counter in Mexico. Ralph was taking what was considered to be a recommended dosage.

The Denver physician who had agreed to administer the experimental program for the independent researchers contacted Ralph. The protocols had been written and the six-week program would start in 2 weeks.

"We'll try the Ribaviron and Isoprinosene for the next couple of weeks," Ralph said, "but when the experimental medication is ready, I'm going to try that. Who knows? It could work. It sounds promising."

"Can you come in for blood work before we start? We have to establish a baseline," he said.

"Sure...when do you want us there?" Ralph responded.

"Tomorrow 10:00 AM."

"We'll be there!"

Ralph had looked forward to this with anticipation. The doctor was going to explain how this new medication would work. Ralph and one other unidentified person would be the only two on the program.

"What if it works? Wouldn't that be something if this was a cure?" he said to Bev when he hung up the phone.

The explanation the doctor gave the following morning was logicial.

"It could work," R.P. said to Bev as he pushed Ralph's wheelchair from the office.

The ride to the doctor's office had upset Ralph. He was nauseous and miserable through the presentation. The doctor attempted to address him on several occasions but he sat with his eyes closed, his head bowed. He did not respond. It was a disappointment to the doctor. He remembered Ralph's keen interest and easy comprehension.

"I'm going to find out about that medication the French have developed at the Louis Pasteur Institute in Paris," Bev said. "They've been doing a lot of AIDS research over there and they just might have something. They're calling it HPA 23."

She contacted the French Consulate in Colorado, who referred her to the French Attaché in Los Angeles. She was given the number of the Pasteur Institute in Paris. They had no positive successes with the medication, but might have something to report in the future.

The voice on the television was familiar, and Bev glanced up to see a face she could not recognize at first sight. "It's Rock Hudson" she thought, "he looks like Ralph." She phoned Rachelle, "Are you watching 'Dynasty'?"

"No."

"Tune in and call me back."

When Rachelle called back, she spoke with disbelief. "Rock Hudson looks just like Dad. I'll bet you anything he has AIDS."

"I thought the same thing," Bev said, "I didn't realize there was a characteristic look with this disease, but now I'm beginning to wonder..."

"Dad didn't resemble Rock Hudson before; what is it that makes them look alike now?"

"There is something about his mouth and jaw, maybe the clenching of his teeth....I don't know."

"I think that's what it is - Dad holds his jaw rigid like that too."

"I hope we're not falling into thinking that just because we're surrounded by this disease everyone else has it too."

"I don't think so, Mom."

"Let me tell you a silly thing that happened last night. I was sitting in the family room; Daddy was upstairs in bed. I heard something like an explosion. I thought it came from the kitchen but I couldn't find anything out of order. I stood looking up the stairs afraid to go up for fear of what I might find. I know Daddy has been discouraged but I didn't think he would do anything like that. I finally got the courage to go upstairs. I peeked into the bedroom and he was sleeping quite peacefully. All night I wondered what that was."

"Did you ever find out?"

"Yes," Bev laughed, "this morning I found a puddle of water on the kitchen floor. The cap from a bottle of club soda bottle blew off in the bottom of the cabinet."

Ralph complained of a pain in his right shoulder. He could only sleep in one position. "It feels kind of like pleurisy," he said.

Dr. Fraser recommended a chest x-ray. "Mrs. Newman, your husband has a partially collapsed lung. I think he should go into the hospital. We should do a bone marrow on him."

"For how many days?" He doesn't like being in the hospital, you know."

"I know. It would be 3 days at the most."

"I'm giving him those experimental medication injections now. How will that be handled?"

"I'll let the people at the hospital know so you can continue. How is that going, by the way?"

"Pretty good, I guess. We haven't seen any sign of improvement yet. I just want to stay with the schedule as it was set up. It's the only way we can tell if it's doing any good."

Laurie brought Jeffrey with her when she came to Denver in April. She was distressed by Ralph's noticeable decline.

The night before Ralph entered the hospital for tests, Laurie tucked two-year-old Jeffrey in bed and said, "You go to sleep now, Grandpa is asleep and we don't want to disturb him."

Laurie joined Bev for coffee at the kitchen table and within a few minutes Jeffrey slowly walked out on to the balcony where Ralph had delivered his "papal" address. Laurie looked up from the table and said, "Jeffrey, you get back in bed and be quiet now."

He turned and went back to bed only to return to the balcony a few minutes later, his natural surprised expression amplified by fear, "Papa! Papa!" he cried pointing back toward Ralph's bedroom.

Bev and Laurie hurried up the stairs. Ralph lay in the middle of the bedroom floor struggling to get up.

"I was going to the bathroom...." he said almost apologetically.

"What happened?" Bev asked.

"My left leg just went numb and it was like it wasn't there."

"Are you hurt?" Laurie asked, Jeffrey peeking from behind her.

"No, I just want to go back to bed."

"Jeffrey told us that something had happened to you," Bev said after Ralph was settled in bed.

"He did?" Ralph said, indicating surprise and pleasure. He reached out to touch Jeffrey's hand. "You're a good boy," he said smiling with appreciation.

The next day at the hospital as Bev entered the waiting room, Laurie said, "Oh, Mom, he has lost so much ground since I saw him in November."

"I know Laurie, I just hope they can find something to treat this time."

"Why does he roll his eyes back like that? That scares me. It seems like it is related to the central nervous system but I have no idea how."

"This is so frustrating. No one can tell us what is going to happen, and then when something happens, nobody can tell us why it has happened."

"What kind of tests are they doing on him this time?"

"One thing they are planning to do is an adrenal function test. He seems to have all the classic symptoms of adrenal insufficiency. They are also going to do a bone marrow, a chest x-ray and then the usual lab work."

"What about the experimental medication? Is he going to continue on that while he is in the hospital?"

"Yes, I'll continue to give him those shots. It is a 6-week program and we dare not miss one day. I've already taken it and put it in the refrigerator at the hospital. I'll give him that shot tonight."

Rachelle and Jim were returning from a 10-day vacation in Norway on the day Ralph was discharged. They went directly to the hospital.

In just 10 days there had been a marked change. Ralph's words were slurred and he was too weak to open the gift they brought him. His once expressive blue eyes were gray – almost uncomprehending.

"What happened to Dad while we were gone?" Rachelle asked Bev when they were alone.

" 'Chelle, I don't have a good explanation for what has happened to him this past week but it could be related to the mistake that was made in administering the experimental medication."

"What?!! What do you mean 'mistake in administering his medication'! Do you mean in the hospital?"

"Yes, here in the hospital. You knew I was giving him those daily injections of experimental medication. Well, when he was hospitalized I brought the medication and put it in the refrigerator. Then, two days ago, when I went to get the bottle from the refrigerator. It was gone! I asked the attending nurse where the bottle of medication was and she said the doctor had taken it. Pressing further, I found that a doctor had come in to do the adrenal function test, thought it was the cortisol he needed and injected the entire bottle into Daddy's vein."

"Oh! For Christ sake, Mom! That was to be injected into his muscle – ½ cc daily! No damn wonder he looks so bad. What was in that crap anyway?"

"The doctor administering the program doesn't think it should be harmful."

"Sure! How the hell does he know!?"

" 'Chelle, we'll probably never know what effect that had on him. He tried to get out of bed to go to the bathroom and fell again. His left leg seems to go numb. You remember when he fell so hard on the patio last summer...."

"What are we going to do?"

"What can we do? R.P. and Laurie and I were here all day while the second adrenal function test was done. R.P. was in the room this morning when the bone marrow test was performed. One thing we know, we can't let anything like this happen again. He is far too sick for any more bungling."

Rachelle sat alone in the waiting room after Bev left. She thought of the way her Dad had greeted her when she walked into his room. "Hi, Pooch." It was a term of endearment for her alone. It never failed to generate a flood of warmth. He had called her "Pooch" or Poochie Pie" since before she could remember.

"I don't want to bring him back here ever again," she thought. Tears filled her eyes at the thought of Brian. "He is 9 years old and he has been so close to Dad. Brian's interest in electronics, computers and engineering is because of Dad. There will never be anyone to fill the void in Brian's life if - I'm afraid to think about it now."

"Let's not bring him back here, Mom," Rachelle said as they left the hospital, "not ever again!"

Chapter Twenty-Five

The physician who administered the experimental medication called late that afternoon. "We must have another blood sample to complete our study."

Bev responded with polite impatience, "Ralph is far to sick to ride across town."

"If it is all right with you, we can come to your house."

"That's fine if you want to do that."

That night Ralph began gagging in his sleep. Bev was frightened... she held him repeating over and over, "You're going to okay, baby... you're going to be okay."

When the gagging stopped, Ralph fell back on the bed and lay in a deep sleep.

The following morning the two doctors arrived carrying a small open cardboard box containing the paraphernalia to draw Ralph's blood.

"Guess doctors don't carry black bags anymore," Bev thought as she showed them to Ralph's bedroom.

"Good morning, Mr. Newman," the doctor said as he entered the room, "Do you know who I am?"

Ralph looked at him with glassy eyes and smiled but did not respond. He wasn't sure. He couldn't remember.

The doctor introduced himself and his assistant. They chatted as they drew the blood directing remarks to Ralph that did not require his response.

As the doctors were leaving, Bev asked them hesitantly - nervously, "What is going to happen?" The gagging the previous night had frightened her. It seemed vaguely like what she imagined a seizure would be like.

".....Well..uh..he won't remember that I was here and he isn't going to get any better," the doctor replied.

"I know – but what will happen?"

"Oh, he will just go to sleep someday and not wake up. But you should not be here alone. Get someone to stay with you."

"I will ... I will," she said, thinking more about his answer to her question than his suggestion.

A few days before Ralph's 56th birthday, Dr. Fraser called. "Mrs. Newman, I have the results of the bone marrow test...the news isn't very encouraging. We have found a mycobacteria in the bone marrow. With this development I have to tell you that the next few weeks are going to be very difficult and the chances of Ralph making it through are slim. There is experimental medication we can start him on....it could help. I should have it in a few days. I'll let you know."

After Bev hung up the phone, she brushed her hair back from her forehead, stared at the ceiling momentarily and then dropped her head to the table. She had feared a call like this one. Now it had come.

" 'Chelle would you pick up Daddy's medication before you come over tonight? Dr. Fraser just called and said it was in." Bev knew Rachelle would be over for Ralph's birthday.

"This will be a nice evening for Dad," Rachelle thought, as she drove toward her parents house. She was pleased with the gift she had bought for her Dad. It had special significance. She turned her head to catch a glimpse. It was still in the back seat, neatly wrapped with pretty paper and tied with a blue ribbon. "He'll like it," she thought, "it's not a big gift, but I'm glad I thought of it. He'll remember my junior high school musical – 'Toyland'." The words from its title song....."once you cross its borders, you can ne'er return again" had brought out a gentleness in him. It had pleased her. Later that evening, after her performance, he'd said, "When I heard those words, I realized my Poochie Pie had crossed that border and it made me sad."

"Sometimes I wish I was back in Toyland," she thought as she approached the subdivision. "I wish things were the way they used to be. Dad was invincible then."

She reached down in the seat beside her for the medication as she drove into the driveway. She carefully picked up the gift from the back seat and dashed into the house. "Mom! Dad! I'm Here. I have Dad's new medication."

" Bring it up 'Chelle. Daddy's awake."

"Hi Pooch," Ralph said as she kissed him and wished him a Happy Birthday.

"I brought you a birthday present but you have to take your medicine before you open it," Rachelle teased.

He took his medication willingly and tugged weakly at the blue bow.

"Here, let me help you," Rachelle said kneeling beside his bed.

"It's a music box, Dad. Can you guess what it plays?"

Ralph shrugged and slowly shook his head, a hint of a smile present.

Rachelle wound the music box smiling as she watched his reaction when it began playing 'Toyland'.

"Oh, that's nice, I've always like that song," Ralph said, his works flat and lifeless.

Rachelle hoped she would see an indication that he remembered but only the twinkle in his eye conveyed that possibility. She put the music box on the headboard, brushed his hair back and kissed his forehead. Her face hardened as she thought with a sad smile, "It's true – you can ne'er return again."

The results of the bone marrow test alarmed the family. Steve, Kathy and Laurie drove to Denver the day after Ralph's birthday. Laurie brought Paula with her and Steve and Kathy wanted him to see their miracle baby after the precarious pregnancy and the cytymegalovirus scare. Rachelle BreAnn was a perfectly normal, healthy baby and Paula was thriving.

Ralph was scheduled for another transfusion. Steve, Laurie and Kathy would have an opportunity to ask questions of Dr. Fraser. They would be there to help Bev make sure everything went smoothly.

As the nurse bustled about the room preparing Ralph for his transfusion, Steve reviewed Ralph's hospital records. The night after the erroneous experimental medication injection, Ralph had fallen getting out of bed and injured his knee. A splint was put on his knee and he was tied in bed.

"Nobody said anything to me about a knee splint or tying him in bed! God! I wish I had stayed with him that night!" Bev said as she and Steve stood outside Ralph's room reading the record.

"I wonder what else went on," Steve said.

A male nurse approached them, whipped the chart out of Steve's hand and as he walked away said, "A doctor on the sixth floor needs this record."

Bev and Steve were puzzled then angry. "What the hell does he mean, 'a doctor on the sixth floor needs this record' – the patient is here!" Bev said in exasperation.

Steve, Kathy and Laurie requested a conference with Dr. Fraser. He tried to be mildly encouraging while remaining truthful. "Your father is very frail – it is possible that the medication for the bone marrow mycobacteria will be effective. We just don't know."

"Have you identified the mycobacteria?" Steve asked.

"No. It really doesn't make any difference – this is the only treatment available."

"Do you know why he rolls his eyes back like he does?" Laurie asked.

"That is probably from the central nervous system involvement. He has had other subtle symptoms in the past – you did know that, didn't you?"

"Yes, we did," Kathy said, "but do you know what is causing the central nervous system problems?"

"No...this is something that happens frequently with AIDS patients. We don't know why."

The conference was discouraging.

After they returned home, Kathy asked Bev, "Have you thought about moving Dad's water bed downstairs?"

"I've thought about it and I think we should. It would be so much easier for me to get Daddy in the car. He likes to go out for lunch and has to go to the doctor so often."

"We could do that this weekend while Steve is here."

"I don't think I would like having my bed downstairs," Ralph said

Kathy was persuasive. "That way Mom can help you out in the family room to sit by the fire and watch television."

"And she can help you to the car when you want to go out for lunch," Laurie said.

After Ralph was settled in his waterbed that evening, he still had reservations. "I don't know if I'm going to like it down here. I like sitting at the coffee table with Mom – I like our bedroom." It wasn't the relocation of the waterbed he protested, it was what the action signified.

Laurie looked around her parent's upstairs bedroom and was drawn to her Dad's collection of Edgar Cayce books. His interest in the subject had intensified her own. She leafed through several of Ralph's Edgar Cayce books. Each one bore evidence of being read thoroughly.

One in particular caught her eye because a page was deliberately creased in half at the title 'Finding an Outer Partner'. She flipped to the last page and saw the words written by Ralph's well-disciplined hand, "Obviously done months ago," she thought. She bit her lip and blinked back tears as she read –

BEVERLY,

I WILL WAIT FOR YOU BEYOND –

SO THAT WE CAN GO ON TOGETHER.

LOVE YOU FOREVER,

RALPH

"I won't show this to Mom...not now anyway," she thought. She placed the book carefully back in the headboard then took a moment to regain composure before going back downstairs.

Ralph smiled as Kathy and Steve entered his downstairs bedroom with Rachelle BreAnn.

"Hey this is pretty nice having your bed down here closer to your red chair and the kitchen," Steve said.

"Yes, I suppose it is," Ralph answered with distraction. He brightened when he saw Rachelle BreAnn, "That's a good lookin' baby you've got there Kathy, even if she does look like Steve." Ralph said, winking at Steve. "Take good care of those babies. Your kids are the only thing you'll leave on this earth that's worth a damn."

Chapter Twenty-Six

Three days later Ralph would not respond to anyone. His eyes were open but he would not speak. Dr. Fraser advised bringing him into the emergency room. It was 8:30 in the evening.

"I think you should call an ambulance," Bev said, "because we don't know what's wrong and he is so weak."

"Please, no sirens," Laurie said, when she made the call.

"We'll be right behind you, Dad," Kathy said as Ralph was carried out through the garage by the ambulance attendants.

"Mom, you go ahead with Dad in the ambulance, I'm going home to get Janet and we'll be right over," R.P. said.

On the way to the hospital the ambulance attendants gave Ralph oxygen. After 20 minutes he was responding to and understanding their questions.

"Mr. Newman, why wouldn't you speak to us before?"

"Because.....I didn't want to," Ralph responded

Laurie and Kathy, with their two babies in strollers, Rachelle, R.P. and Janet were in the emergency room waiting area. "I find it curious that the oxygen affected him so favorably," R.P. said.

"He could have a recurrence of pneumocystis," Laurie said, "Or whatever it is, he might benefit by having oxygen available to him at home."

"I don't like bringing Dad back here," Rachelle said peeking through the small window in the door leading to the examining rooms.

"What's going on in there?" Kathy asked as she adjusted the blanket over the baby's stroller so the overhead lights wouldn't shine on her face.

"Mom is just talking to the doctor."

"Excuse me, 'Chelle," R.P. said, brushing past her, "I'm going in there."

Laurie came into the waiting room, pushing Paula in her stroller. "I wish this kid would go to sleep," she said.

"Here – Let me push her around," Rachelle said taking the stroller from Laurie, "You go in there and find out what's going on."

Laurie walked in on Bev and R.P.'s conversation with the doctor, "...and we'll be doing a chest x-ray," the doctor said.

"Pneumocystis doesn't show up on chest films," Bev said as they walked together to the lobby.

"Mrs. Newman, we are professionals here. If you would just let us do our work now, we'll let you know what we find." Motioning toward the waiting group, "Why don't you tell your family to go home and get some rest. This could take hours. There is no need for all of them to be here; there's nothing they can do."

"Hah!" Kathy said, "We're staying right here until we find out what's wrong."

"That's right!" the others chimed.

When the doctor came into the waiting room 45 minutes later he addressed Bev as if she were alone in the waiting room.

"Mrs. Newman, we're going to need your consent to do a spinal tap."

"Have you done arterial blood gases?" Laurie asked trying to catch his eye.

"Yes," he replied without turning to look at her.

"Mrs. New...."

"What were the results?" Laurie interrupted forcing his attention.

"Normal."

"Will you be culturing for cryptococcus when you do the spinal tap?" Laurie asked quickly before he had a chance to ignore her again.

"Are you a doctor?" he asked, sarcastically.

"No, I'm not."

"A nurse?"

"No, Med Tech."

The doctor turned to Bev, shutting out everyone around him, "I'll bring the consent form for you to look over."

R.P. came into the waiting room as the doctor left. "That catheterization was so painful for Dad," he said as he slumped into a chair. Holding his head in his hands, "I was wishing I hadn't talked him into having it done."

"You had no choice. It had to be done but I know how you feel R.P.," Bev said laying her hand on his shoulder.

"Now they're going to be doing a spinal tap. I hope that isn't as painful," R.P. said.

The doctor came out with periodic reports, addressing Bev exclusively – deliberately ignoring the other family members.

R.P. turned his head, his eyes following the doctor as he left the room. As the door closed, R.P. jumped to his feet, "I'm going in there to find out what's going on."

He found Ralph in a half sleep, lying on a hard narrow cot, with a soiled pad. The floor was littered with debris, including a bloody needle. Stepping into the hall, he hailed a nurse. "What's this?!" he said gesturing toward the debris, "Do you see that bloody needle?"

"Oh – yes, that shouldn't be there."

"I didn't think so!"

The babies lay sleeping in their strollers as the family waited for results of the spinal tap.

At 5:00 AM the doctor walked into the waiting room and stood directly in front of Bev to exclude the attention of the others. "The results of the spinal tap were negative. There is something wrong in his urinary tract – he does have a catheter in but you can take him home and bring him back tomorrow to see a urologist."

Bev turned her head slowly, looking at him with incredible astonishment, "You've got to be joking."

"No, I'm not. We've found nothing we can treat and we can't keep him here."

"Let me understand this - you're telling me, after I brought this sick man into the hospital by ambulance and you've put him through a full night of testing including a spinal tap, that I should take him home with a catheter and bring him back tomorrow to see a urologist?"

"That's right."

"You're crazy!"

"Mrs. Newman, there is nothing we can treat."

"Okay, I understand that, but couldn't you keep him here until he can be seen by a urologist?"

"I don't know if seeing urologist is going to do any good – and then there is the expense of keeping him here..."

"Expense! Expense?! This disease has already cost the insurance company $150,000. Do you think they or I would flinch at one more day in the hospital?"

"I think you should discuss that with Mr. Newman."

"Oh, for Christ sake! Be reasonable! Ralph couldn't care less what this is costing at this point."

"We can't keep him here," he shrugged.

Her look was as cold as his words. "Take the catheter out! I'll take him home," she said. Then turning to Rachelle, "Call an ambulance. Let's get him out of here."

The nurse brought Ralph into the waiting room in a wheelchair with a urinal bottle in his lap.

Laurie grabbed the urinal bottle. "Could we please have a plastic bag for this?"

"Sure, I'll get one for you. I'm sorry, I know how sick Mr. Newman is. He's been in so often some of us feel we know him. I guess there's something about hospital policy..."

As the ambulance attendants took Ralph out the door, his family filed out behind him. "Hospital policy?" Laurie said spitting on the floor defiantly, "That's what I think of your hospital policy!"

Chapter Twenty-Seven

The family reconvened at home on the patio, while Ralph rested in his waterbed after the long ride home in the ambulance. When Bev went in to get a fresh pot of coffee, R.P. said, "We're going to have to persuade Mom to take Dad back to the Mayo Clinic. I know Dad would insist on it if this were one of us."

"I agree!" Kathy said. "We can't take a chance on something like this happening again. Dad is too sick."

Bev came out onto the patio and began pouring coffee.

"Did you see that doctor's socks?" Kathy said, "They were Mickey Mouse socks – they actually had a big picture of Mickey Mouse on them."

Everyone had seen the doctor's Mickey Mouse socks. The shared laughter served to buffer their anguish. Bev passed a plate of pastry around, "Danish anyone?"

"Sit down Mom. We want to talk to you." R.P. said ignoring her offer.

Bev looked around the table. She knew whatever R.P. wanted to talk about had been discussed in her absence. R.P. was speaking for the group.

"I think we should take Dad back to the Mayo Clinic," he said, "We're not getting any answers here – last night was an example."

Bev looked at R.P. and then out across the back yard. "He is so weak," her voice shaking, "I don't think it's wise to take him so far away from home. Why don't we let him make the decision?"

R.P. responded with a tinge of annoyance, "Mom! We can't let Dad make that decision now – he's damn near incoherent!" He drew back momentarily, sorry for his words. He knew how it hurt his mother to hear them. He also knew they would regret it if they didn't pursue every available avenue. It was risky and the chances of getting help were slim. "But we have to try, Mom."

"I know, R.P., but getting him there could be very difficult. Even by plane it is an exhausting trip."

"Don't worry about that," Rachelle said, "I'll take an early flight in to Rochester and arrange for the ambulance, hotel rooms and anything else you need...."

R.P. interrupted, "...and I'll go with you to help get him on and off the plane."

"You'll make it Mom," Kathy said, "You never know, they might be able to help him. If anyone can, they can."

"We'll help you get Dad ready to go," Laurie said.

They pleaded their case and sat by quietly waiting for Bev's response.

"Okay," she said nodding her head, "I just hope everything goes smoothly." Pushing her chair back from the table she said, "I'm going to check on Daddy."

Ralph was awake. "I have to get dressed and go to the doctor to have these tubes taken out this morning," he said in a much stronger voice than she thought possible.

Weakness swept through Bev as she stood by his bed. The evidence that Ralph was suffering brain damage was mounting. Temporary? Permanent? Progressive? Extent? No one knew.

She sat on the edge of his bed holding him in her arms. "You don't have any tubes. They were taken out at the hospital last night," she said matter-of-factly, trying to hide her concern. "R.P., 'Chelle and I are taking you to the Mayo Clinic tomorrow."

"That's nice, Mom. Where are the kids? I want to see them."

Ralph's spirits were lifted. They hadn't given up on him and if they weren't giving up, neither was he.

It was a warm sunny day when the ambo-cab pulled into the cul-de-sac. Bev looked out at the driver pulling the ramp down and unloading the wheelchair. Suddenly she wished they had taken Ralph to the airport in the car.

Ralph waved to Kathy and Laurie as he was rolled through the side door. He was pleased to be going back to the Mayo Clinic. Just 2 miles into the 20-mile trip to the airport Ralph began to vomit.

"Please stop!" Bev said, "I have to help him."

The driver pulled to the side of the road. "This could be a very long trip," Bev thought as she wiped Ralph's mouth.

R.P. and Janet met them at the airport.

R.P. lifted Ralph from the wheelchair into his seat on the plane and within a few hours they were in Rochester.

Rachelle was at the Rochester Airport when they arrived. The ambulance was waiting; the hospital was expecting Ralph. Their motel reservations were made.

Ralph was settled comfortably in his hospital bed within the hour.

"He's getting the attention, consideration and care we wanted for him," Rachelle said as she, R.P and Bev ate dinner late that night.

"I knew this was the right thing to do. Even if they don't find anything they can treat, we will never be sorry we did this," R.P. said.

"You're probably right," Bev said, "But one step at a time. I'm just glad we got him here."

In addition to routine testing, a complete neurological workup was done.

"We'll have to do another bone marrow test. We don't rely on test results from other clinics," the doctor said, "and we want to test for cryptococcus. That wasn't done."

For the first two days in Rochester, R.P. was in more discomfort and pain than Ralph. The stress of previous months had taken its toll. He lay in the motel room suffering with a severe case of hemorrhoids.

"R.P., you have to have something done," Bev said, "You can't let this go on. I'll ask the emergency room at the hospital if they can take care of you this afternoon."

"Okay, I hope they can do something."

R.P. was admitted that afternoon for treatment of what was diagnosed as thrombosed external hemorrhoids. As he lay on the cot in the emergency room, he overheard the hospital personnel speaking in hushed tones. He picked up... "Newman".... "AIDS".

"Ah, that could be why they've drawn six vials of blood," he thought.

"You might have me confused with my father," he said to the nurse, "His name is the same as mine only I'm the junior. We both live in Littleton, Colorado and have our health insurance through the same employer. My father has AIDS. He is on the fifth floor."

R.P. was given a room on the fourth floor with the number of his room differing from Ralph's by one digit. The climate was right for confusion.

That evening as Rachelle and Bev waited outside, R.P. had surgery. They were there when the nurse brought him out pale, perspiring and exhausted.

Through the evening Rachelle and Bev kept Ralph informed of R.P.'s status – he was doing fine. They also kept R.P. informed as to Ralph's status.

Since being admitted to the hospital, Ralph had not shown any signs of confusion. He conversed normally with family, nurses and doctors. Ralph's day had been remarkable. He felt good and expressed deep concern for R.P.

"Are you going to stay with me tonight?" he said to Bev.

"I think I'll go back to the motel. 'Chelle and I haven't had anything to eat, but I'll be back early in the morning."

"Aw, Mom, you and I used to sit and talk till the wee hours of the morning," he pleaded.

"You'll be going to sleep soon," she said kissing him on the cheek, "this has been a long day."

Ralph watched them leave. He felt lonely.

"Have you ever been to Colorado?" he asked the nurse.

"No, I haven't Mr. Newman, but I would like to visit there some day. I understand it's beautiful."

"You are welcome to stay with us anytime. We have a big house and there is a little creek that runs nearby....the fishing is good too."

"I would like to see it. Thank you for the invitation," she said, "I might just do that."

When Bev entered his room the next morning he was unresponsive.

"What is wrong, Ralph?" Bev asked. "Tell me if you are hurting. Has the doctor been in? Did they give you an injection this morning?"

Ralph's face flushed, twisting into a deep frown, "Beverly! Leave – me—alone!

For Ralph, this was in uncharacteristic response. He normally liked attention. He drifted into a deep sleep and then into a coma later that day.

A CAT scan revealed an undefined abnormality on the left side of his brain.

"This has happened to other AIDS patients. We don't know why, except that the virus must attack the brain tissue," the doctor said, "I'm sorry we don't have more answers for you."

"Would you call the Louis Pasteur Institute in Paris and ask them about their experimental medication HPA 23?" Bev asked.

"We sure can do that."

"Also, there is a doctor in California who has been doing some research with white cells that has shown promise – could you contact him too? I have the telephone numbers for both." She said flipping her book open and reading as he wrote.

A few minutes later Dr. Morrow entered the room. "I'm so sorry that I didn't come in yesterday," he said, "I understand Mr. Newman was doing just fine then."

"Yes he was. We don't know what happened," Bev said turning to Ralph, "Ralph it's Dr. Morrow. Can you squeeze my hand?"

There was no response.

"Kathy and I'll be leaving on the morning flight for Rochester. Grandma is coming with us," Laurie said when Rachelle called to give her and update.

After hanging up the phone Laurie stood at the kitchen sink, looking through the window as one of Ralph's favorites songs played softly in the background. "Fight, Dad! Fight!" she cried as she tried to overcome the immobilizing effect of Rachelle's report.

They were in Rochester by the next afternoon. Laurie sat at the end of Ralph's bed, her head resting on her arms. "I'm praying for a little miracle here," she said. She'd seen patients in Ralph's condition. They rarely regained consciousness. "I wish I could play some music for him," she thought as the picture of him recording their old favorites flashed through her mind. She smiled to herself remembering the times they clashed over her choice of music when she was a teenager.

"You can play that garbage music on my stereo – I'll make that concession but you won't play it when I'm in the house!" he'd said. He'd taught her to appreciate good music and she was grateful.

Her fists clenched in frustration as she remembered his words – 'can you help me?'. "If I'd only known! Why didn't the Center for Disease Control warn people. They were getting reports on this disease almost two years before Dad had surgery. We could have had blood donated for him. How can our government allow an industry to function without full disclosure of the dangers associated with their product?" She lifted her head to look at Ralph. Nothing had changed. "All I want is a little miracle, Lord."

The doctors were not encouraging. "We can't tell you how this is going to go. I'm sorry there's nothing we can do. I've contacted the Pasteur Institute and it will be some time before they could accept him as a patient. Then he would have to go to Paris."

Bev shook her head and asked, "And the California doctor?"

"He's at a conference."

"Mrs. Newman, I have to ask you how you want us to handle this. The way things are now, we don't know which way this will go and we must make a decision in advance. Do you want us to use heroic means to keep Mr. Newman alive?"

"Heroic means?"

"By that I mean do you want us to call a....a.....if his heart should stop or if he stops breathing, I must tell you that without your permission we would have to perform some very invasive procedures which would include putting him on a respirator. Truthfully, I don't think you...."

"No, I don't want that – he's been through enough."

"If at all possible, we'll want to take him home"

"I think that's the best thing. Let's hope it works out that way."

Ralph began moving his feet during the night. By midmorning the next day, it was as if he had just awakened from a good night's sleep.

"Hi, I'm thirsty. Can somebody get me some water?" he said to the astonishment of everyone in the room.

"Hi, Dad, how are you feeling?" Laurie said.

Kathy rushed to his bed, "I love you Dad," she said hugging him tightly.

"I'm kind of hungry. How about some tacos?" he said.

"We'll be right back with your tacos," Rachelle said as she and R.P. left the room.

"Look what I brought you," Kathy said handing him a picture of Scotty and Stephanie.

He took the picture, studied it, turned it over, turned it back and laid it on the table in front of him with out comment.

Laurie and Kathy looked at each other. They were confused.

"How about a piece of candy, Dad?" Laurie said placing a wrapped chocolate on the table beside the picture.

He looked down at the table and reached with his thumb and forefinger for the candy, missing by two inches. He drew his hand back studying the table. Again he reached for the candy and missed.

Laurie and Kathy watched, disappointment and hurt evident in their eyes.

"Let me unwrap it for you," Laurie said, as she took the candy from the table, unwrapped it and handed it to him. Ralph had regained consciousness but something was wrong. It discouraged them.

The next morning, when Bev came in to the room, Ralph said, "We're going home today."

"That's right, we are. Just as soon as we have everything ready," Bev said.

"I'll get up and help you load the car," he said.

"No, baby, you don't have to do that. We're going to fly." She said taking his clothes from the closet. "You'll be home in your own bed tonight."

"You're going to need a wheelchair," Rachelle said, "I'll have Jim pick one up and bring it over tomorrow night."

"Thanks, 'Chelle. If everything goes as planned we should be there. I'll be glad to get Daddy back home."

There was no direct flight from Rochester to Denver. Ralph would have to be taken by ambulance from Rochester to the Minneapolis airport. It was there that Laurie, Kathy and Bev's mother would board their plane for North Dakota as well. They said their goodbyes to Ralph as he was lifted from the gurney and strapped in the wheelchair.

He lapsed into a state of semi-consciousness for the remainder of the trip and was unaware that R.P. and Jim carried him into the house and put him in his waterbed that evening.

The following weekend, Rachelle came over to take care of Ralph so Bev could run a few errands.

"Take your time Mom," Rachelle said as Bev was leaving, "I'm planning to spend the night. We'll watch a movie or something..."

"Great 'Chelle, I'll see you later."

Rachelle enjoyed the afternoon alone with her Dad. All went smoothly and Bev returned early that evening.

"How was your afternoon?" Bev asked as she laid her purchases on the counter.

"Gee Mom, Dad seems so weak. Does he still walk well enough for you to help him to the bathroom and out to his chair?"

"Yes, it's been working pretty well. I set the wheelchair by the bed and he clasps his hands behind by neck and then he stands long enough to swing around and sit down. The bathroom is only 10 feet away. I get him out of the bathroom the same way."

"Oh, he's gone downhill so fast."

"I know, 'Chelle, I don't know what to do anymore."

"I'm concerned. Are you sure you can handle this alone?"

"Well, I guess I've just been taking it one day at a time."

Ironically that night as Rachelle was upstairs getting ready for bed, Bev helped Ralph into the bathroom through the standard routine and proceeded to help him from the stool in the usual manner. Ralph clasped his hands behind her neck, stood to do his half turn and his legs both buckled under him. Bev, on her knees, held his torso upright but his legs remained twisted beneath him. His eyes were open in a blank stare. Bev called frantically, " 'Chelle! Help me!"

Rachelle ran downstairs to find them on the floor in the bathroom.

"Oh God! What happened?"

"His legs just buckled!"

The wheel chair still blocked the door and Rachelle pulled it out of the way and knelt beside Ralph. He continued to stare fixedly at nothing.

"Dad? Can you hear me?"

No response.

"Ralph," Bev gently shaking him, "Ralph."

No response.

"Now what do we do?" Rachelle asked.

"You hold the wheelchair and I'll try to get him into it."

The wheelchair would not fit through the bathroom door. Rachelle pushed it up to the door and leaned over the back to hold it steady as she tried to help. Bev wrestled with Ralph trying to lift him from the floor. She backed toward the door still holding Ralph and ended up sitting in the wheelchair with Ralph on her lap. Ralph was still limp and unresponsive.

"This isn't going to work Mom!"

"Obviously!" Bev snapped. "Oh, God."

"If you can ease him back on to the floor I'll get this wheelchair out of here and get a blanket."

"Okay, let's lay him down."

"Do you think we should call R.P.?"

"No, let's just get him lying on the floor first, then we can figure out what to do."

Rachelle spread the blanket on the floor and helped ease Ralph on to it – his eyes still blank and staring.

"Let me get him something to drink," Rachelle said.

She quickly returned with a glass of water and a straw and dribbled a few drops at a time into his mouth.

"That's good – a few drops at a time. I'm afraid he'll choke." Bev said, exhausted and bewildered. "I think we can get him into bed if we each take one end of the blanket and slide him into the bedroom."

"Okay, let's go!" Rachelle said.

They lifted him onto the bed and sat with him until he was asleep.

"I'll go fix us some tea," Rachelle said, "I think we both could use it."

'Chelle, I don't know what I would have done if you hadn't been here. How did I happen to end up sitting in the wheelchair anyway?"

Shaking her head Rachelle said, "I don't know Mom, it was all so bizarre! But, I have to say you and I put on a 'Fric and Frac' act if I ever saw one!"

"No kidding!" Bev said as they both laughed through their tears.

Chapter Twenty-Eight

"Are we going to meet R.P. for lunch today?" Ralph said smiling at Bev.

Bev was encouraged to see Ralph responsive and alert. Much of the time, when he sat in his chair, she felt like a little girl having a tea party with a doll. She helped him into his chair, carried on a one-sided conversation and then helped him back to bed.

"Yes, we are. This is going to be a nice day." She said as she combed his hair.

"Make me look like Jeffy," he said playfully, "even Toms says we look alike."

Going out for lunch was a rare occurrence. Ralph spent more and more time in bed. He even objected when Bev told him he would need another transfusion.

"Let's just skip it this time. I don't like that long ride."

"Would you be more comfortable in your patio lounge chair in the back of the suburban?"

"I guess we could do it that way, Mom, but I don't think these transfusions are doing any good. I lay there for hours with that needle in my arm – then I come back home and feel just as bad but I'll go if you say so."

"R.P. is going along to help. We're going to make it as easy for you as we can."

He reluctantly agreed to compromise.

R.P. backed the suburban up to the emergency room door. He and Bev carried Ralph in. He was transfused in his lounge chair, returned to the suburban and his waterbed with minimal trauma.

Laurie and Kathy were uneasy with the reports of Ralph's condition. In early May they drove to Denver bringing their "stroller babies," Paula and Rachelle BreAnn. When they arrived, Bev discussed the possibility of contacting a hospice nurse.

"She will come over a few times a week and help care for Daddy. We can call her in an emergency if the doctor is not available."

"Mom, I think it would be a good thing," Laurie said, "Do you want me to call her?"

"We have to have approval from Dr. Fraser first."

"Why?" Laurie asked.

"Because hospice care is only afforded to people who have six months or less to live."

"What do you mean?" Kathy said – angry and distressed.

"Kathy, we know Daddy is very sick – things could still turn around – but for now I think Dr. Fraser would approve it."

Laurie contacted the hospice nurse who came over the next afternoon. She was a kind, capable lady. She had shared hopelessness with families before. She knew how they felt – she knew what to say.

The preliminary discussion took place in the living room.

"There are some things I feel that patients shouldn't hear," she said, "but I would like to meet Ralph."

He was seated in his red chair in the family room. She presented herself to him in a friendly and understanding manner. His response was cold and distant. He sensed something he didn't approve. He wondered what they had to say that he couldn't hear.

"We've had other AIDS patients under our care," she said trying to break through, "I know you don't feel good – some of the people have a lot of trouble with thrush. Have you had that problem."

"Yes," said Bev breaking the uncomfortable silence.

"There is a new medication that seems to be working well for most people."

"Oh really, what is it?" Bev asked, "We should get some of that – it might make him feel better."

Ralph looked straight ahead. Bev's apparent enthusiasm irritated him. Without changing his expression, in slurred speech he said, "Probably tastes like cat piss!"

As the nurse left, Bev thanked her and offered a vague apology. She patted Bev's shoulder and said, "Honey, you call me if I can help."

"We're going shopping today," Laurie said after coffee and Danish with Ralph. "Tomorrow is Mother's Day, Dad. What kind of card do you want us to get for Mom? Funny or serious?" Laurie asked.

"Oh, a fairly serious one," he responded weakly.

Bev stopped them as they were leaving. "I'll pay you, but please pick up something for me from Daddy. I know he'd feel bad if he didn't have something to give me tomorrow."

"Do you need anything else?"

"Yes, would you pick up some club soda – Daddy has to have his fizz."

When Bev finished giving Ralph his bath she set Paula in her walker on Ralph's bed. They entertained each other while Bev cleaned the bedroom.

"This is one way you and I can both stay out of trouble," Ralph said to her.

"Now is there anything else I can get for you before you take your nap?" Bev asked.

"Yes. How about a plain fizz -- and a plain hug."

"In that order?" she laughed.

"I'll take the hug first."

"How are you doing?" Bev asked as she entered Ralph's room early that afternoon. He did not respond. He began to gag and vomit. Fear gripped her as she quickly turned him on his side, holding his head and repeating over and over, "You're going to be okay, baby - you're going to be okay."

She wished desperately for the kids to come home. Ralph was in a state of semi-consciousness while she changed the sheets and his pajama top.

It was late afternoon when Kathy and Laurie came bustling in with their packages. "Is Dad awake?"

"No, he isn't. I'm really glad you're home. He had a bad gagging spell again - like the one he had in the night a couple of weeks ago. Only this time he vomited. He's been sleeping ever since."

Laurie and Kathy were anxious to show Ralph the gift they had bought for him to give to Bev. "This is it!" They said when they saw the red dress. "Dad loves to see Mom wear red."

An hour after the spirited shopping spree, they moved like robots. R.P. and Bev gently slid Ralph onto his lounge chair into the suburban and headed for the hospital.

"I'm going with you," Kathy said.

" 'Chelle's at the farm. I'll call her and be right behind you," Laurie said.

" 'Chelle – Dad had a convulsive seizure about an hour ago. He's in a coma. We're taking him to the hospital right now."

"Which hospital?"

"The same one."

"Oh, God!"

"I know, but the doctor told Mom they would admit him directly."

Turning abruptly from the phone, Rachelle said, "Jim! We have to go home right now!"

"But 'Chelle, that's a 150 mile drive, it's after 10:00 pm and the kids are tired. Maybe we should wait until morning."

"Okay Jim but if I don't get there in time, I'll never forgive you!"

The melodramatic performance might have been amusing under different circumstances. Within 15 minutes they were on the road to Denver.

Rachelle rushed breathless into Ralph's room as the surgeon walked out.

"What's going on?"

"Dad has a collapsed lung. They just inserted an aspirator tube in his rib cage," Laurie said, "and they're giving him medication intravenously to stop the seizures."

"Don't touch him or talk to him," the nurse said, "it excites the nervous system and that will cause more seizures."

R.P. sat quietly beside Ralph's bed, his hand close to his Dad's. He reached out to touch but not touching the long slender fingers so thin now. "He put is garnet ring away months ago. The garnet ring," R.P. thought, "a college graduation gift from Mom. He was so proud of it."

R.P. recalled Ralph's words: "I want you to have my ring, R.P." he'd said when he put it away. The subtle implication of the words weighed heavily on R.P.'s mind now. When he was a teenager R.P. had watched with fascination as the ring danced over the yellow crosshatch pad while his Dad wrote, sketched, drew, taught. He was always teaching. R.P. had often watched the light rays reflect from it and let its hypnotic effect blot out the words his Dad was saying – the lesson he was trying to convey. "The lessons! Why didn't I listen closer? What did I miss?" R.P. thought. "Dad had no father to admire, to teach him lessons, to take him hunting. He had no pattern to follow. He cut his own pattern. By his own admission, there were rough edges but it was there for me to follow, to modify."

Now R.P. felt a new responsibility. He wanted to make the garnet ring dance. He wanted to fascinate a son with the light rays. He wanted to be admired by a son. He wanted to walk surefooted as if he mentally wrote an equation for each step – as his Dad had.

Anger swept through him. He wanted to punch someone. He wanted to make someone suffer as his Dad had suffered these past two years. He wanted revenge for the times his Dad sat listening to blood banking officials denying that this could happen. "I don't think we should get alarmed," they'd said, "more people die from bee-stings than have died from transfusion AIDS." He wanted revenge for the thoughtlessness! He wanted revenge for the reckless abandon!

The brilliant mind that made it possible for the garnet ring to dance with a unique style had faded so quickly. The slender fingers lost their dexterity. His vision was failing. He never said he couldn't read – he hoped they wouldn't notice. R.P. would never see the garnet ring dance through a child's eyes again. He wanted revenge.

He looked at his Dad and suddenly felt overwhelming guilt for his anger. Bits and pieces of the Saturday morning lectures came back.

"Whatever happens to you happens for a reason. Look for the lesson to be learned. The problems you encounter are not nearly so important as how you handle them. Life is never easy. You have to be tough but you must try to understand."

"I'm going to try to be tough, Dad," he thought, "I'm going to try to understand. It won't be easy but I promise you, I'm going to try."

Kathy had seen Ralph's seizure. His room was darkened to reduce all stimuli. "He's so helpless," she thought. She'd stood by the bassinet of her infant son, Scotty, three years earlier and had been overwhelmed by his dependence, his helplessness. She remembered her pledge, "This little boy will have the tenderness, love and attention Dad longed for as a child."

Now she was grateful for the maturing process. It permitted her to understand what she, as a child, had considered "Dad's unreasonable behavior." She was familiar with his emotional make up. She had inherited it. When they were happy, the whole world knew it and when they were displeased, everyone suffered.

Her Dad's pursuit of purpose in the mid-seventies had led to revelations resulting in a mellowing and contentment in him she never thought possible. She was glad he had those years of contentment. As it emerged, no one appreciated the gentle nature more than she.

"Dad really had his life together," she thought, "He and Mom should have had these years to enjoy together, instead of this struggle for survival in a web of unknowns." She listened to his labored breathing and the gurgling aspirator tube. The sight of her mother out of control shocked her. "This shouldn't have happened," she thought, "Dad is only 56 years old. Their lives are wrecked!"

She jumped to her feet, tossing her long dark hair away from her face. "I'm going to kill the person responsible for this," she thought, running to the door, opening it hard against the wall. Her rage was uncontainable as she ran through the corridor to the waiting room.

"I'm going to kill the person responsible for this! My Dad is being murdered!" she screamed kicking the metal trash container across the waiting room and tipping over chairs in her way, convulsing in tears in her mother's arms.

The nurse followed her calmly straightening the chairs and putting things back in order. Quietly understanding, "I don't blame you," she said.

"Now, this is Mother's Day," Laurie said, "I know this has probably been the worst day of your life but why don't you open the gift from Dad?"

Bev opened the box with the red dress. One of Ralph's great pleasures was giving gifts. She leaned over his bed and touched her lips lightly to his cheek. "It's beautiful....I love you."

Ralph never saw the red dress.

Midmorning the next day two young doctors walked into Ralph's room. "Mrs. Newman, your husband has a condition called progressive multi-focal leukoencephalopathy. The white matter in his brain is being affected by the virus – or a virus. Few viruses can penetrate the blood-brain barrier – this one can."

"Is there anything we can do?"

"There is no effective treatment."

She had never seen the two young doctors before. She never saw them again.

"Get your book, Laurie!" Bev said.

Moments later Laurie reported, "There is a medication used to treat progressive multi-focal leukoencephalopathy but it has toxic side effects. I don't think it would work now."

"Thanks Laurie, we tried," Bev was resigned. "Why don't you kids run home and check on the babies. You've been here all night. I'll stay with Daddy now."

She was alone in Ralph's room. She smiled sadly, "This is the way we started," she thought as she moved around the end of the bed, "alone." She tenderly brushed a wisp of hair from his forehead as she spoke to the deep recesses of his mind.

"Oh, my baby, I love you so much. I know you're hurting and I just want you to know, if you want to go, it's okay. We have four kids you can be proud of. We were good together – we were a good team." She brushed the back of her fingers across his cheek and bent forward to touch her lips to his forehead. "If you want to go, it's okay – we'll meet again."

"You've been brave soldiers," Bev said as the tiny platoon prepared for retreat.

Never before had she appreciated them more than at that moment. "Ralph is right!" she thought, "Your kids are the only thing you're going to leave on this earth that's worth a damn!"

***

And so we run before the sun
This mystery to unfold
For he has gone beyond the sun
And the pattern we behold
Is one unfinished tapestry
Dark threads among the gold.

Rachelle Newman Mollohan

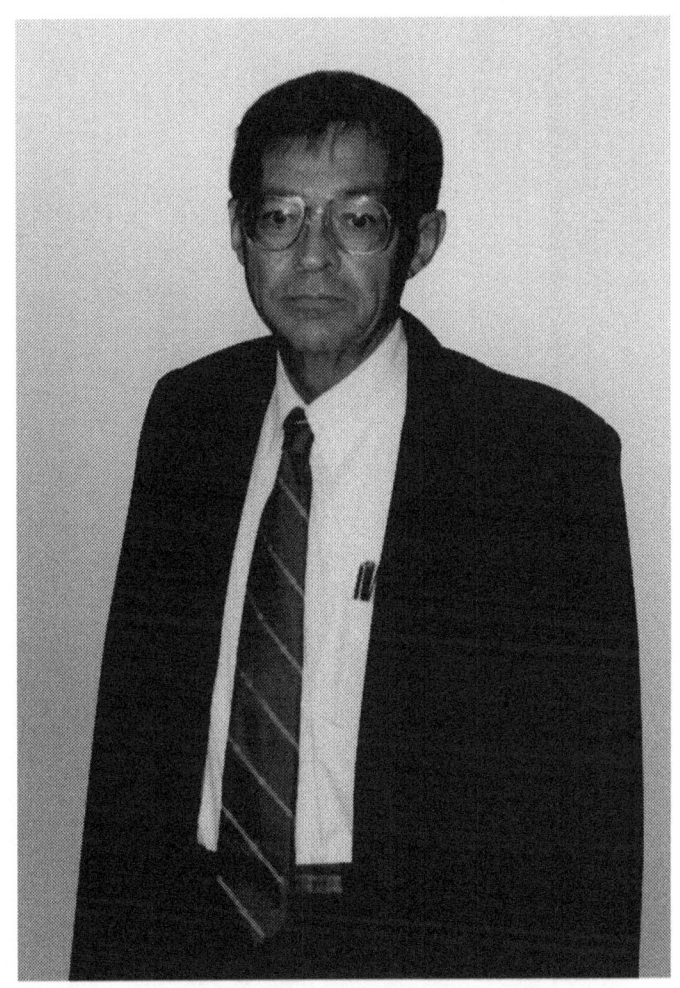

Ralph P. Newman
October 1984

Epilogue

My husband, Ralph P. Newman, died of transfusion associated AIDS at 3:33 PM on Tuesday, May 14, 1985.

I have chosen to share the details of his illness, and the emotional trauma to my family, in an effort to promote greater understanding and awareness of AIDS patients and their families. To permit the tragedy or Ralph's death to become a mere statistic in a dusty file bin would be an injustice to him and to those who can learn from his experience.

Our search for treatment or cure is over. Only the haunting questions remain. How could this contamination of the blood supply have gone undetected for so long? Have the FDA, the Department of Health and Human Services and the legislators assumed a responsible role in regulating the blood banking industry to prevent the spread of AIDS? What can we do to provide support to AIDS patients and their families?

We felt that if - through talking to people, speaking to groups, sharing information we could prevent one person from contracting AIDS, our efforts would not be in vain.

The details of Ralph's experience with AIDS have been recounted in newspapers, magazines, television programs as well as clubs and church groups.

R.P. prepared overhead slides for a presentation to members of his church.   Rachelle, R.P. and I were invited to speak at a Kiwaniis breakfast and I spoke to a gathering of preschool mothers.

As a result of an invitation to participate in the NBC *Today* show, I had the opportunity to meet the mother of the little boy who died of transfusion AIDS. She was the only member of our "support group" at that time.

While the Colorado legislators were debating AIDS legislation, we were asked by the sponsor of the bill to testify before a Senate Committee. R.P., Rachelle and I entered the small hearing room with the hope that our testimony would help pass the bill into law. However, as is the case with so many AIDS bills, controversial measures are attached and the bill becomes over-encumbered. It did not pass.

On May 16, 1985, two days after Ralph's death, it was disclosed in the New England Journal of medicine that one of Ralph's blood donors tested positive for the HTLV-III antibody and was a member of a high-risk group.

In compiling information to substantiate our lawsuit, we found that the contaminated blood was transfused to Ralph in the form of fresh frozen plasma and that one of the donors of fresh frozen plasma was on unspecified medication with a temperature of 95.7 degrees F.

The responses from the physicians we consulted regarding extreme subnormal temperatures in a blood donor were many and varied – "The donor could be a mouth breather," "The donor may have been drinking ice water," "It must have been a faulty thermometer," "The tech read the thermometer wrong," But all agreed that if this was a valid temperature the donor was a very sick man.

The Merck Manual (the most widely read medical text in the world) defines accidental hypothermia as "an unexpected fall of body temperature to 95 degrees F." The manual also states that "Phenothiazine treatment, congestive heart failure, starvation, ketoacidosis, pulmonary infection, sepsis, brain injury, any sort of immobilizing illness predispose to hypothermia."

In a meeting with the field representative of the FDA, I was informed that there is no minimum temperature guideline in blood banking regulations. There is, however, a stipulation that a qualified donor should have a normal temperature; anything below 99 degrees F. is normal.

I wrote to Dr. Frank Young, the Commissioner of Food and Drugs at the FDA in Rockville, Maryland. In his response to my query he stated....

"The Food and Drug Administration regulates the blood banking industry and while current regulations stipulate that a qualified donor should "have a normal temperature', no standards have been set for subnormal temperatures because there is no known communicable disease for which a subnormal temperature is the sole symptom. A high temperature can be a reliable indicator of infection, and the American Association of Blood Banks has specified a maximum donor temperature to guard against the risk of infection. However, that group's standards do not include a low temperature limit."

If this were an industry without a history of disease transmission, the rationale that "no known communicable disease for which a subnormal temperature is a sole symptom" would be acceptable. However, screening procedures in blood banking have never been considered diagnostic tools, only indicators of potential health problems.

Establishing that the HTLV-III positive donor was the same donor as the one with the 95.7 degree temperature was essential in pursuing our lawsuit.

Following are excerpts from our letters of appeal to the U.S. Department of Health and Human Services, the Centers for Disease Control and the Colorado State Health Department:

- We are targeting only the HTLV-III positive donor.

- Is the donor with the suppressed immune system the same donor who tested positive for HTLV-III?

- We are requesting disclosure of the temperature of the HTLV-III positive donor at the time of donation and/or his birth date.

- We have NEVER requested, nor are we now requesting, the identity of the donor.

- In reviewing the donor cards supplied by the blood center, we find that of the four donors of fresh frozen plasma, one had a temperature of 95.7 degrees F. at the time of donation and was on unspecified medication.

All governmental agencies responded by denying any information associated with the positive donor.

Further hampering our legal action was the fact that the disease was not recognized by the Centers for Disease Control when Ralph was transfused. At the suggestion of our attorney, we voluntarily withdrew our lawsuit in January 1986.

In spite of the growing concern for the safety of the nation's blood supply, the screening test for donated blood did not become **compulsory** by FDA regulation until February 1988 – three years after it became available. Although the incidence of transfusion AIDS is far greater than originally stated, there is no nationwide systematic method for testing blood recipients. Those who receive contaminated blood are innocently exposing their wives, husbands or sexual partners.

Senator Armstrong of Colorado was sufficiently concerned for the safety of the blood supply to enter the following into the Congressional Record on April 10, 1987. " On December 9, 1982, the Centers for Disease Control in Atlanta announced it was investigating the cases of 20 children with AIDS symptoms. One child, who died at the age of 20 months, has received numerous blood transfusions for an unrelated condition. The CDC reported, 'This and continuing reports of AIDS among persons with hemophilia raise serious questions about the possible transmission of AIDS through blood and blood products."

At the end of the same month, a Newsweek magazine article on AIDS told readers that...

"The Department of Health and Human Services is expected to convene an advisory panel soon to assess the role of blood transfusions in spreading the disease...But public health officials warn against undue alarm, especially since only one case has been strongly linked to transfusions."

Dr. Harold Jaffe of the Centers for Disease Control was quoted as saying, "The risk to the general population is quite small."

During the following year other health officials made similar statements.

On July 14, 1983, the New York City Health Department, the Council of Hospital Blood Bank Directors of the Greater New York Region, Inc. and the Greater New York Hospital Association issued a statement asserting: "Physicians can reassure their patients that the community's blood supplies are not considered a source of the spread of AIDS."

In a July 25, 1983 U.S. News & World Report article, Los Angeles Red Cross administrator Norm Kear claimed: "The odds are 10 million to 1 against someone getting AIDS through a blood transfusion." The magazine explained to readers that -- So far, only one person – among the 3 million Americans who receive blood every year – is thought to have contracted AIDS from a routine blood transfusion; an infant in San Francisco.

On September 15, 1983 the United Press International wire service reported that American Red Cross President, Richard F. Schubert defended his agency's blood collection methods by saying the risk of getting AIDS from a blood transfusion are "infinitesimal," according to a United Press International report of that date.

On October 16, 1982, according to an AP wire story of that date, Dr. Edward N. Brandt, an assistant Secretary of Health and Human Services said, "Let me make it clear, the blood supply of the nation is safe. I have no concern and would not be afraid of receiving blood anywhere in the country."

On November 2, 1982, the Associated Press reported on a news conference held by American Blood Banks. Dr. John Bove of Yale School of Medicine, a spokesman for the association said the risk of contracting AIDS from a transfusion was one in one million.

On the same day, the Washington Post reported that –

Federal Health Officials and blood bank leaders meeting here (New York) today said the American blood supply is highly safe. The chance of getting AIDS from a blood transfusion is still very small.... less than one in a million.

My point is very simple. Today experts are saying something quite different. Of the estimated 9 million Americans living today who received transfusions during the period of concern. 1978 to 1985, public health officials now say as many as 12,000 may have been infected with the virus. This is a far cry from 1 out of 1 million, which would be 9 people not 12,000.

The reasoning in all this is not to criticize errors in estimates or even the failure to understand all the dangers. AIDS is a relatively new disease. Our health professionals have learned a great deal in a very short time. But along the way, all of the rest of us who are not experts have been treated to pronouncements issued with an unwarranted air of certainty. My preference is for more caution and less dogma.

As we should have learned from our experience with the nation's blood supply before 1985, categorical denials or assertions about AIDS are off the mark. The public is wise enough and compassionate enough for an open and full discussion of this epidemic and that may mean challenging the prevailing wisdom about it. After all, the prevailing wisdom has been wrong before.

Tributes

Ralph's roots were in North Dakota. His final resting place is there on the prairie where the geese fly over in the fall and the winds blow free.

At the close of the funeral service, Tom, in his small single-engine plane with Jeffrey at his side, flew over the gravesite – tipping his wings in final salute.

Although Ralph had courted atheistic beliefs during his college days, his search for purpose resulted in a deep faith in God that sustained him through his last days. Ralph had his own unique style and we wanted his marker to reflect that special quality.

After consulting several sources, we found an epitaph from scripture:

Love – As Above, So Below

This is inscribed on Ralph's marker along with his name in his own handwriting and a permanent ceramic picture from a photograph taken by Kathy in her front yard. If he were looking down at our efforts, I think he would approve.

On Flag Day 1985 Laurie and Kathy with the Battle Hymn of the Republic playing in the background lowered the tattered flag from

Polaris Park in Minot, North Dakota and raised a new one in memory of their father.

On December 25, 1986 - a final tribute from his beloved grandchildren: The International Star Registry re-designated Star Number Centaurus RA 11h37m25sec, to the name of Ralph Paul Newman. Henceforth, this star will be know by his name, is permanently filed in the Registry's vault in Geneva, Switzerland and is recorded in a book which is registered in the copyright office of the United States of America.

I CAN FLY, YES I CAN FLY

There once was a time
I questioned life around me
But now I have wings,
I know the answers well.
Life is for the learning,
It teaches lesson hard.

Now I see the rainbow,
After the storm is passed.
I feel the colors within,
So bright, so bold so fast.

Soaring above the heavens,
Like an eagle when it flies,
I've come to take you with me,
Now close your eyes.

Do you see the colors? Do you see the light?
It isn't long before I come back to you in flight.
I can fly. Yes, I can fly, over mountains, over seas
To catch the rainbow now that I am free.

I've set the course before me,
I am searching for the key
Working to show you
That there is no guarantee.

You reach out to touch me,
You falter but yet you go.
To catch the rainbow,
And maybe tomorrow you will know.

Jenene Kelley
(Close family friend)

The wind is whispering through this tree
Do not despair, his soul is free.

Yet, the time was so brief since he sat on that porch tread
And ate of Grandma's sugar bread.

The crocuses and deer he found upon this place remain
To hear the meadowlark's refrain.

He climbed so many hills to gain success,
And found a love to share his happiness.
The evil thing that through his veins did flow,
And snatched his body from its goal,
Did not gain – for upon this earth he will remain
Far longer than this flag unfurled
Or marker with his name.

This is the final hill,
The highest peak he can ascend.
From here his spirit shines among the stars
And meets the rainbow's end.

The birds fly by and tip their wings
Farewell, my friend.

To Sonny Boy – Ralph
Who took me by the hand,
Buried my pennies
And tied me to trees.

Colleen Alme
(Ralph's cousin)

Dear Reader,

It is my hope that Ralph's story has broadened your scope of understanding. There have been significant advancements in research and education since Ralph was diagnosed. The information available today enables us to take a knowledgeable stand on AIDS – knowledge is our only tool against hysteria. A rational approach will make it possible to extend a warm and loving handclasp to the afflicted with out fear.

And what of self-preservation? The few simple recommendations for disease prevention are easy to follow. Read them carefully and keep them close at hand.

If you are concerned about receiving blood, donate your own prior to surgery if possible or if you wish, select your own donors.

If you are among the afflicted and have questions that cannot be answered by your local physician, contact the Centers for Disease Control in Atlanta, Georgia or the National Institute of Health in Rockville, Maryland. You will find the people in these institutions compassionate, dedicated individuals who work day and night to unlock the mysteries of this unprecedented epidemic.

If you are caring for a family member with AIDS, seek a support group and consider contacting hospice for assistance. Then resolve to live each day to the fullest for the time you bear the burden will be brief.

Look forward – the answers are there – If we search for them, work for them, tomorrow we'll know.

Sincerely,

Beverly M. Newman

Beverly M. Newman

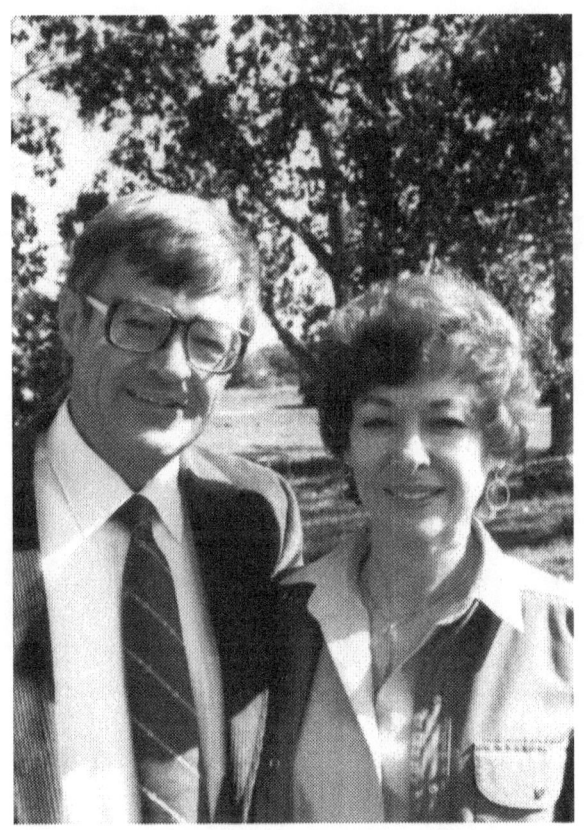

Ralph P. Newman   Beverly M. Newman
April 1929 – May 1985   February 1933 – July 1998